Pharmanual

A comprehensive guide to the therapeutic use of ®Trasicor

AF863306

Editor
Stevo Julius, University of Michigan,
Ann Arbor, Mich., USA

35 figures, 8 tables, 1984

KARGER

Basel · München · Paris · London · New York · Tokyo · Sydney

Pharmanual

A comprehensive guide to the therapeutic use of

1 **Cefsulodin**
VI + 94 p., 28 fig., 1 cpl., 36 tab., 1980. ISBN 3-8055-1024-X

2 **Aminoglutethimide**
2nd, revised edition
VI + 162 p., 59 fig., 2 cpl., 40 tab., 1982. ISBN 3-8055-3452-3

3 **Cefotiam**
VI + 182 p., 6 fig., 52 tab., 1983. ISBN 3-8055-3694-1

4 **®Trasicor**
VIII + 115 p., 35 fig., 8 tab., 1984. ISBN 3-8055-3836-7

National Library of Medicine, Cataloging in Publication
A Comprehensive guide to the therapeutic use of ®Trasicor
editor, Stevo Julius. - Basel; New York: Karger, 1984.
(Pharmanual; v. 4)
1. Oxprenolol - pharmacodynamics 2. Oxprenolol - therapeutic use
3. Cardiovascular Diseases - drug therapy
I. Julius, Stevo II. Series
ISBN 3-8055-3836-7
WI PH321T v.4 [QV 150 C737]

Drug Dosage

The authors and the publisher have exerted every effort to ensure that drug selection and dosage set forth in this text are in accord with current recommendations and practice at the time of publication. However, in view of ongoing research, changes in government regulations, and the constant flow of information relating to drug therapy and drug reactions, the reader is urged to check the package insert for each drug for any change in indications and dosage and for added warnings and precautions. This is particularly important when the recommended agent is a new and/or infrequently employed drug.

Printed in Switzerland by Thür AG Offsetdruck, Pratteln
ISBN 3-8055-3836-7

Contents

III. Oxprenolol (®Trasicor) – Scientific Profile

Foreword

When confronted with a new pharmaceutical product, or with updated information on an existing drug, the physician is most often left to rely on a complex of charts, scales and diagrams in order to determine the applications of the product, judge its effectiveness, and ensure optimal therapeutic results. The *Pharmanual* series has been created as an alternative source of information. Published in the form of compact guidebooks, these manuals are written and edited with a practical orientation, offering the physician clear directions concerning the therapeutic possibilities of selected drug products.

Each *Pharmanual* incorporates extensive research organized into three main sections. The first focuses on discussion of the relevant disease entities. The second presents critical reviews of the treatment alternatives now available to patients and physicians.

The goal of ensuring optimal therapeutic results with a product is served through a third section where clinical and pharmacological information is presented in the form of extensive in vivo and in vitro data. The final part of this section offers clinical guidance and advice as prepared by physicians who have themselves had intimate experience with the particular pharmaceutical product.

With these important information needs satisfied in a concise, expert text, the *Pharmanual* series will be a valuable aid in determining how products can be most beneficially applied toward improved management of human disease. This is especially important when updated information on existing products can improve their use for the benefit of the patient.

The Publishers

Introduction

Since *Ahlquist* postulated the theory that two types of adrenoreceptors mediate the different and frequently divergent types of responses to sympathetic stimulation, the doors have been opened for a new, growing field. The development of various sympathetic receptor antagonists leads to further refinements in our understanding of the physiology of the autonomic nervous system. Thanks to this phenomenal pharmacologic expansion we now know that there are beta-1- and beta-2-receptors, that alpha-receptors in the brain decrease central sympathetic discharge, that there are alpha-1- and alpha-2-receptors and that depending on their location in the sympathetic synaptic cleft there is further functional differentiation amongst the alpha- and beta-receptors. The availability of pharmacologic antagonists lead to the purification and isolation of receptors, to assessments of their affinity, and to actual determinations of their numbers. Were these the only achievements facilitated by the development of sympathetic antagonists, they would suffice. The sympathoadrenoreceptor antagonists, however, have become indispensable therapeutic tools in modern medicine. The proliferation of the field has been phenomenal; scores of new compounds are reaching the market, and new indications for their use are constantly being discovered, placing a burden on practicing physicians. It simply is difficult to keep up with the field.

Against this background, a volume on oxprenolol could not be credibly produced, unless attempts were made to assess the entire field of beta-adrenergic blocking agents and to describe the diseases in which their use has proved to be useful. We will also cover the diseases in which the final proof is not yet available, but in which there is strong evidence that the treatment may be useful. Working from an agreed-upon outline, the four authors in four different countries produced a remarkably consistent manuscript. At no time did the Editor have to settle conflicting views. Apparently all of us interpret the existing evidence the same way. There are, however, differences in individual styles, attesting to our different backgrounds. This is how it should be; books are not written by committees, but by individual authors.

It is our hope that we have provided the reader with the appropriate background and sufficient facts to assess the pharmacologic properties and clinical usefulness of oxprenolol.

Stevo Julius

I. The Heart at Risk

Hypertension

Stevo Julius

Ann Arbor, Mich., USA

Epidemiology

An elevated blood pressure is a worldwide problem [13]; the prevalence of clinical hypertension ranges between 5 and 20% of the adult population. This statement immediately raises the question of definition: what is hypertension? The blood pressure in populations is distributed in a bell-shaped fashion. Therefore, any cutoff point between normal and abnormal readings will be arbitrary and can only be set by convention. When a variable is continuously distributed, the standard method for defining pathology is to consider as abnormal those individuals whose values are below or above two standard deviations of the population's mean. However, the blood pressure issue is more complex for two reasons: (1) blood pressure readings tend to vary and (2) there is a continuous relationship between blood pressure level and mortality; a higher blood pressure, even within the normal range, carries a higher mortality than a lower normal reading. Consequently, definitions of hypertension always specify conditions of measurement and usually choose a blood pressure level at which mortality is above the average for the entire population. This blood pressure level is substantially lower than two standard deviations above the mean. The World Health Organization [18] defines hypertension as a single, sitting or recumbent blood pressure exceeding 160/95 mm Hg. Values below 140/90 mm Hg were considered normal. A later report [17] stated that readings between 140/90 and 160/95 mm Hg below age 30 should be considered with suspicion. Borderline hypertension is a term now generally used for individuals whose readings fall between clearly normal and definitely elevated.

If one is to obtain comparable data, the blood pressure measurement technique must be standardized. The proper technique is well described in a recent publication of the American Heart Association [3]. In short, the width of the inflatable bladder should be 40% of the circumference at the midpoint of the forearm, and the length of the bladder should be twice the recommended width. The patient should be comfortably seated with the arm slightly flexed and with the entire forearm supported at heart level. Measurements should be taken at least once on both arms. The pressure in the cuff should be inflated 30 mm Hg above the point at which the radial pulse disappears and then released at a rate of 2–3 mm Hg/s. The fourth phase (muffling of the Korotkoff sound) is taken as the diastolic pressure.

The WHO has a typical epidemiologic definition of hypertension. It is based on large blood pressure surveys (hence one reading) and on the prognostic significance that such readings have on average longevity. However, a clinician requires a different definition. A physician needs to know the individual and not the average prognosis in order to decide whether a patient requires antihypertensive medication. Whereas the average mortality risk is excessive for the population whose one reading is 160/95 mm Hg, many such individuals are at lesser risk. These are the patients whose blood pressure subsequently becomes normal. This is a frequent event. The author has shown that in only 30% of patients with slightly elevated readings were the hypertensive readings maintained when subsequent repeated values were averaged [8]. Consequently, a better blood pressure description is required for the clinical definition of hypertension [7]. The major issue in clinical practice is whether the antihypertensive treatment prescribed will effectively prevent future complications in an asymptomatic patient. For all intents and purposes, to a clinician hypertension is the lowest blood pressure level at which antihypertensive treatment has been shown to improve a patient's prognosis. Fortunately the question of efficacy of antihypertensive treatment has been thoroughly investigated [1, 6, 16]; all studies were based on a clinical definition of hypertension, e.g., repeated blood pressure readings before a patient was enrolled in the study. There is a consensus that when the average repeated diastolic blood pressure exceeds 95 mm Hg, antihypertensive therapy is indicated and saves lives. Therefore, the diastolic blood pressure in a patient with clinical hypertension must always exceed 90 mm Hg, and the average of at least two readings taken on separate days must be over 94 mm Hg. The Hypertension Detection and Follow-up Program Cooperative Group [6] suggests that treatment is useful in all patients who maintained a diastolic blood pressure over 90 mm Hg on two repeated occasions, even if the average was below 95 mm Hg. However, the study is fraught with methodologic problems, and the results cannot be extrapolated to general medical practice [4].

Hemodynamics of Hypertension and Its Consequences

It is noteworthy that all clinical studies use diastolic blood pressure as a measure of the severity of hypertension, despite clear evidence that elevated systolic blood pressure is an equally strong predictor of future cardiovascular morbidity [10]. The preference for diastolic blood pressure is rooted in misconceived 'physiologic' thinking. Hemodynamically the blood pressure is a product of cardiac output and vascular resistance. In established hypertension, the cardiac output is normal and blood pressure elevation is due to a high vascular resistance. The diastolic blood pressure is thought to better reflect this high vascular resistance, since the systolic blood pressure can be high in conditions with low vascular resistance (exercise, hyperthyroidism, A-V shunts). This thinking is incorrect because a vascular resistance can be substantially elevated with very little elevation in diastolic blood pressure. A change from the recumbent to the sitting position causes a 27% increase in total peripheral resistance, while the diastolic blood pressure is barely elevated [6, 9]. It is incorrect to assume that systolic blood pressure elevation is innocuous and has no effect on cardiac performance or on any other aspect of cardiovascular function [5].

The consequences of hypertension are of two types: pressure-related complications and complications due to the premature development of atherosclerosis. The cardiac sequelae of high blood pressure are left ventricular hypertrophy and congestive heart failure, whereas the cardiac manifestation of premature atherosclerosis is coronary heart disease. It is important to differentiate between these two types of blood pressure related cardiovascular complications, as they respond differently to antihypertensive treatment. Blood pressure lowering is very effective in reducing pressure-related cardiac morbidity. For example, in the Veterans Administration Study [16] of mild hypertension (diastolic 90–114 mm Hg), after 40 months of follow-up, there were no cases of congestive heart failure in the group on active antihypertensive treatment, whereas 5.6% of those on placebo developed congestive heart failure. Congestive heart failure is a direct consequence of the increased afterload on cardiac muscle. The afterload is a function of the

Table I. Coronary risk factors in LVH-negative nonsmokers versus LVH-negative smokers [from ref. 3]

Cholesterol level mg/100 ml	Systolic blood pressure, mm Hg											
	105		120		135		150		165		180	
	non-smokers	smokers	non-smokers	smokers	non-smokers	smokers	non-smokers	smokers	non-smokers	smokers	non-smokers	smokers
Glucose intolerance absent												
185	2.5	3.9	3.0	4.6	3.6	5.5	4.3	6.6	5.2	7.9	6.2	9.3
210	3.0	4.7	3.6	5.6	4.4	6.7	5.2	7.9	6.2	9.4	7.4	11.1
235	3.7	5.6	4.4	6.7	5.2	8.0	6.3	9.5	7.4	11.2	8.8	13.2
260	4.4	6.8	5.3	8.0	6.3	9.5	7.5	11.3	8.9	13.3	10.5	15.6
285	5.3	8.1	6.4	9.6	7.6	11.3	9.0	13.4	10.6	15.7	12.5	18.3
310	6.4	9.7	7.6	11.4	9.0	13.5	10.7	15.8	12.6	18.4	14.8	21.4
Glucose intolerance present												
185	3.3	5.0	3.9	6.0	4.7	7.1	5.6	8.4	6.6	10.0	7.9	11.8
210	3.9	6.0	4.7	7.2	5.6	8.5	6.7	10.1	7.9	11.9	9.4	14.0
235	4.7	7.2	5.7	8.6	6.7	10.2	8.0	12.0	9.5	14.1	11.2	16.5
260	5.7	8.6	6.8	10.2	8.1	12.1	9.6	14.2	11.3	16.6	13.3	19.4
285	6.8	10.3	8.1	12.2	9.6	14.3	11.4	16.7	13.4	19.5	15.7	22.6
310	8.2	12.2	9.7	14.4	11.5	16.9	13.5	19.6	15.8	22.7	18.5	26.2

LVH = Left ventricular hypertrophy.
Numbers represent the probability (per 100) of developing coronary heart disease in 6 years according to specified characteristics.

physical properties of the heart (chamber size and wall thickness) and of total resistance to the systolic ejection of blood. This resistance to ejection does not depend only on mean arterial pressure, but is substantially influenced by properties of the vascular system. A less compliant arterial system will substantially increase impedance to arterial ejection [14]. A decreased compliance of blood vessels is invariably associated with an increased systolic blood pressure. This increased systolic blood pressure requires that force be generated by cardiac muscle, thereby substantially increasing external cardiac work. Since both systolic and diastolic blood pressure reflect increased impedance to cardiac ejection, it stands to reason that both should be given equal priority in antihypertensive treatment.

The relationship between elevated blood pressure and the subsequent development of coronary atherosclerosis has been well established. However, contrary to pressure-related complications of hypertension (stroke and congestive heart failure), this atherosclerotic manifestation of long-standing hypertension is not prevented by antihypertensive medication. For example, in the Veterans Administration Study [16], the incidence of myocardial infarction was, in fact, slightly higher in the treated compared with the placebo group. The inability to prevent the development of coronary heart disease with antihypertensive treatment raises interesting questions. The linear relationship between coronary risk and blood pressure level suggests that blood pressure at least is a quantitatively aggravating factor in the natural history of coronary heart disease. Why then does blood pressure lowering not prevent this aggravation? A real possibility is that some antihypertensive agents, while they lower blood pressure, may in their own right speed the development of coronary heart disease. Particularly suspect in this regard are the diuretics which increase such coronary risk factors as blood lipids, glucose, and uric acid. The recent suggestion, from the Multiple Risk Factor Intervention Trial Research Group [11], that antihypertensive treatment with diuretics may be deleterious, is highly provocative, but the evidence is rather weak.

The last frontier to conquer with antihypertensive treatment is the prevention of coronary heart disease. There is some indication that this may be possible. Monotherapy with various beta-blocking agents has been shown to be effective in preventing a reocurrence in patients who suffered a myocardial infarct [2, 12, 15]. It remains to be seen whether these encouraging results on secondary infarct prevention in nonhypertensive subjects can be confirmed for the primary prevention of myocardial infarct in hypertensive individuals. The question of possible differential effects of diuretics and beta-blockers on mortality and morbidity in hypertension is under scrutiny in Great Britain. The soon-to-be completed Medical Research Council trial may well provide the answers.

Whereas increasing blood pressure invariably leads to a higher coronary risk, the absolute level of risk depends on additional characteristics. Premenopausal women have a lower risk for all complications of hypertension than do men. When hypertension is combined with another risk factor for coronary heart disease, a new profile of coronary risk emerges. An illustration of how four major risk factors for coronary heart disease interact is given in table I. It can be seen that a 50-year-old male in the United States will have a 4.3% probability of developing coronary heart disease, if he has a normal cholesterol level, does not smoke, and his systolic blood pressure is 150 mm Hg. If he smokes, the risk increases to 6.6%. A cholesterol level of 260 will increase the risk to 11.3%.

Clearly, if coronary heart disease prevention is the goal, one must consider risk factors superimposed on an elevated blood pressure. While the scientific discussion about the public health impact of dietary intervention or cessation of smoking continues, the data in table I clearly indicate what needs to be done on a practical level. Whenever possible, while treating hypertension the physician should also encourage the reduction of other coronary risk factors.

References

1 Australian National Blood Pressure Study: The Australian therapeutic trial in mild hypertension. Lancet *i:* 1261–1267 (1980).
2 Beta-Blocker Heart Attack Study Group: The beta-blocker heart attack trial. J. Am. med. Ass. *246:* 2073–2074 (1981).
3 Coronary Risk Handbook: Estimating risk of coronary heart disease in daily practice, pp. 14–15 (American Heart Association, New York 1973).
4 Freis, E.D.: Should mild hypertension be treated? New Engl. J. Med. *307:* 306–309 (1982).
5 Gordon, T.; Kannel, W.B.: Multiple contributors to coronary risk. Implication for screening and prevention. J. chron. Dis. *25:* 561–565 (1972).
6 Hypertension Detection and Follow-Up Program Cooperative Group: Five-year findings of the Hypertension Detection and Follow-Up Program. Reduction in mortality of persons with high blood pressure, including mild hypertension. J. Am. med. Ass. *242:* 2562–2571 (1979).
7 Julius, S.: Borderline hypertension: epidemiologic and clinical implications; in Genest, Koiw, Kuchel, Hypertension: physiopathology and treatment, pp. 630–640 (McGraw-Hill, New York 1977).

8 Julius, S.; Ellis, C.N.; Pascual, A.V.; Matice, M.; Hansson, L.; Hunyor, S.M.; Sandler, L.N.: Home blood pressure determination: value in borderline (labile) hypertension. J. Am. med. Ass. *229:* 663–666 (1974).
9 Julius, S.; Pascual, A.; Sannerstedt, R.; Mitchell, C.: Relationship between cardiac output and peripheral resistance in borderline hypertension. Circulation *43:* 382–390 (1971).
10 McGee, D.: The probability of developing of certain cardiovascular diseases in 8 years at specified values of some characteristics; in The Framingham Study: an epidemiologic investigation of cardiovascular disease, sect. 28, DHEW Publ. No. 74 (New York Academy of Sciences, New York 1973).
11 Multiple Risk Factor Intervention Trial Research Group: Risk factor changes and mortality results. J. Am. med. Ass. *248:* 1465–1477 (1982).
12 Norwegian Multicenter Study Group: Timolol-induced reduction in mortality and reinfarction in patients surviving acute myocardial infarction. New Engl. J. Med. *304:* 801–807 (1981).
13 Paul, O.: Epidemiology of hypertension; in Genest, Koiw, Kuchel, Hypertension: physiopathology and treatment, pp. 613–630 (McGraw-Hill, New York 1977).
14 Tarazi, R.C.; Ferrario, C.M.; Dustan, H.P.: The heart in hypertension; in Genest, Koiw, Kuchel, Hypertension: physiopathology and treatment, pp. 738–755 (McGraw-Hill, New York 1977).
15 Taylor, S.H.; Silke, B.; Ebbutt, A.; Sutton, G.C.; Prout, B.J.; Burley, D.M.: A long-term prevention study with oxprenolol in coronary heart disease. New Engl. J. Med. *307:* 1293–1301 (1982).
16 Veterans Administration Cooperative Study Group on Antihypertensive Agents: Effects of treatment on morbidity in hypertension. II. Results in patients with diastolic blood pressure averaging 90–114 mm Hg. J. Am. med. Ass. *213:* 1143–1152 (1970).
17 World Health Organization: Tech. Rep. Ser. Wld Hlth Org., No. 231 (1962).
18 World Health Organization: Tech. Rep. Ser. Wld Hlth Org., No. 168 (1958).

Stevo Julius, Division of Hypertension, Department of Internal Medicine, University of Michigan Medical School, Ann Arbor, MI 48109 (USA)

Angina pectoris and Cardiac Arrhythmias

Alberto Zanchetti

Milan, Italy

Introduction

With the decline in deaths from infectious and contagious illness, coronary artery disease has become one of the most common causes of death in western societies, being responsible for from 100 to more than 500 deaths per 100,000 population. Now, after many years of a progressively rising rate of coronary deaths, the trend has begun to reverse itself; during the past few years, the mortality rate has been declining. Although these findings are encouraging, the picture is still confused. Figure 1, which summarizes data from a recent report by the National Heart, Lung and Blood Institute [12] shows a marked decline in the number of deaths from coronary artery disease in the United States, Australia, and Israel, but no substantial change in Italy, Czechoslovakia, and France. In other countries – e.g., England, Germany, Sweden, and Poland – the rate is still rising.

If a significant and general improvement in the prognosis of cardiovascular disease is taking place, then physicians as well as investigators have even greater responsibilities. Undoubtedly, the improved prognosis is associated with increased knowledge of the mechanisms and clinical manifestations of coronary artery disease, improved dietary habits, and with the development of more effective pharmacotherapeutic agents. Further and more widespread reductions in the numbers of deaths from coronary disease will depend on the clinician's knowledge of available cardioprotective drugs and their uses in the treatment of angina pectoris, myocardial infarction, and cardiac arrhythmias.

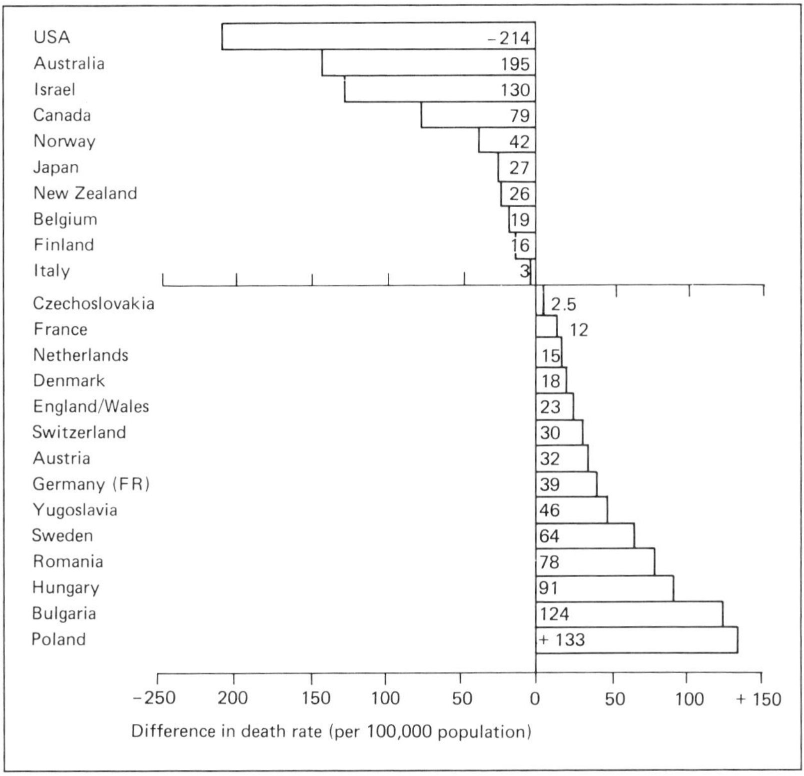

Fig. 1. Trends in mortality from coronary heart disease. Differences in death rate between 1977 and 1969 for males aged 35–74 years in various countries of the world [from ref. 12].

Angina pectoris

Concepts of both the clinical aspects and pathophysiologic mechanisms of angina pectoris have changed considerably in recent years. Today, the once classic definition of angina as recurrent episodes of chest pain due to an increased demand for oxygen by the myocardium is now considered too limited because prolonged electrocardiographic recordings, especially the more extensive use of ambulatory procedures, have shown that the typical changes of angina often occur without pain [15]. Consequently, attacks of transient myocardial ischemia occur much more frequently than clinically overt attacks in many patients. Attention has been focused on spontaneous anginal attacks, i.e., without an effort-induced increment in myocardial oxygen demand. *Guazzi* et al. [4] were the first to show that Prinzmetal's variant angina is usually associated with signs of decreased performance and, therefore, with a reduced rather than an increased myocardial demand, a finding subsequently proved for other types of spontaneous angina. Consequently, angina at rest is caused by a sudden reduction in coronary blood flow and not by an increased demand for myocardial oxygen [2]. This decrease in myocardial blood supply has been shown angiographically to be caused by a sudden and transient block of one of the major epicardial arteries, probably by a vasospasm [11]. The vasospasm may be localized or diffuse, occurs at the site of a severe stenosis or, at times, in angiographically normal vessels, and is usually reversed spontaneously or can be relieved by nitroglycerin or calcium antagonists.

Exactly what causes the vasospasm and whether it is responsible for all cases of angina at rest or whether some other mechanism – e.g., platelet aggregation, microthrombi, etc. – causes the sudden decrease in blood supply to the myocardium must still be clarified.

Classification

Of the current classifications of angina listed in table I the author prefers classification A – exertional angina, angina at rest, mixed angina – because it is based on clinical records of anginal attacks and considers the two different mechanisms leading to transient myocardial ischemia. It is similar to classification B, presented by *Maseri* [10], but emphasizes two opposing pathogenetic mechanisms and assumes that any decrease in coronary blood flow is caused by a primary coronary event, such as a vasospasm. Classification C is also clinically important; it stresses the different clinical courses of angina with time. That is, some patients remain relatively stable, and their angina is mild, while others develop an ingravescent stormy course associated with an increasing risk of sudden death or of myocardial infarction. However, classification C underestimates the useful clinical and pathophysiologic distinction between exertional angina and angina at rest. In the author's opinion, the terms stable and unstable angina define stages of the disease – exertional, at rest, and mixed angina can each run a stable or unstable course. Furthermore, whether unstable angina is associated with an increased mortality risk has been questioned [5], so that a clear distinction between stable and unstable angina may be difficult [1].

Table I. Classification of angina pectoris

A. *Based on clinical pattern and pathogenetic mechanisms*
   (1) *Exertional angina.* Clinically, angina occurs during any kind of exertion requiring an increase in myocardial oxygen demand; it includes angina during muscle exercise, during digestion, during tachycardia, during increased arterial pressure. Pathogenetically, exertional angina is due to increased oxygen demand beyond the limits of a reduced coronary reserve. Anatomically, there are stenotic lesions in one or more coronary arteries. Electrocardiographically, the typical feature is depression of S-T segment.
   (2) *Spontaneous angina or angina at rest.* Clinically, it occurs at rest and in the absence of any sign of cardiac stimulation, without tachycardia, blood pressure increase, etc. Pathogenetically, it is probably due to a sudden reduction in myocardial blood flow without any increase in oxygen demand; it may be due to coronary 'vasospasm' with or without concomitant coronary artery stenoses. Electrocardiographically, there can be either depression or elevation of the S-T segment, the latter pattern characterizing Prinzmetal's variant angina.
   (3) *Mixed angina.* Clinically, episodes occur both during exertion and at rest. Pathogenetically, some episodes are due to increased oxygen demand, others to decreased blood supply. Anatomically, there are usually coronary artery stenoses. Electrocardiographically, the S-T segment is usually depressed during exercise-induced attacks and can be either depressed or elevated in spontaneous attacks.

B. *Based on pathogenetic mechanisms*
   (1) *Secondary angina.* It corresponds to exertional angina and includes all forms secondary to increased oxygen demand.
   (2) *Primary angina.* It corresponds to angina at rest and implies all forms are due to a primary coronary event reducing blood flow, probably a 'vasospasm'.
   (3) *Mixed angina.*

C. *Based on the clinical course*
   (1) *Stable angina.* Angina occurring at fixed work loads.
   (2) *Unstable angina.* Angina of new onset or development of crescendo angina or angina pectoris at rest as well as with minimum exertion. Prinzmetal's variant angina is sometimes included in this syndrome, sometimes classified apart.

Ischemia-Induced Cardiac Arrhythmias

Death due to myocardial ischemia, whether an acute myocardial infarction, angina attack, or an otherwise clinically silent episode, is most often caused by arrhythmias. In recent years evidence has accumulated showing the importance of cardiac innervation – both sympathetic and vagal – and blood-borne as well as local catecholamines in cardiac arrhythmias induced by acute myocardial ischemia [9].

According to *Pantridge* [14] signs of autonomic disturbance appeared in most patients within 30 min from the start of acute myocardial infarction; signs of excessive sympathetic activity were more frequent with anterior infarctions, whereas vagal overactivity was most frequent with inferior infarctions. *Malliani and Lombardi* [7] and *Malliani* et al. [8] provided experimental evidence that cardiac sympathetic activity can be augmented reflexly during myocardial ischemia by cardiocardiac sympathetic reflex excitation. The afferent branch of these reflexes is represented by fibers originating from the heart and travelling in the cardiac sympathetic nerves. Thus, excitation of sympathetic cardiac afferents could affect the heart by affecting sympathetic outflow to the heart.

The sympathetic hyperactivity induced in experimental myocardial ischemia and clinically observed in acute myocardial infarction could in principle have opposite effects. On one hand, sympathetic hyperactivity could contribute to the maintenance of normal ventricular function through increased contractility, thus opposing ventricular dilatation and vagally mediated depressor reflexes. On the other hand, increased sympathetic activity can deleteriously alter the balance between oxygen supply and demand, especially in the myocardium at risk.

Mechanisms Responsible for Cardiac Arrhythmias

Classic models (fig. 2) have shown that the reentrant mechanism is activated in an area of slow conduction with transient or permanent unidirectional block. Ischemia and catecholamines cooperate in generating slow cardiac potentials and, therefore, play an important role in the genesis of reentrant arrhythmias. Potassium leaks out of the myocardial cells, and during ischemia, it accumulates in extracellular space. The consequent

---

Fig. 2. Schmitt-Erlanger model of reentry. The shaded area exhibits unidirectional orthograde block and slow retrograde conduction and generates reentry.

Fig. 3. Model of Na^+ and Ca^{++} channels in the sarcolemma, and mechanism by which norepinephrine (NE) can induce slow potentials. h represents the inactivating and m the activating gate of the Na^+ channel, d and f the activating and, respectively, the inactivating gate of the Ca^{++} channel. Left: normal resting potential and normal action potential. Center: ischemia with potassium offlux, reduced resting potential, and slow potential. Right: combination of ischemia and catecholamines generates a large slow potential [from ref. 16, with permission].

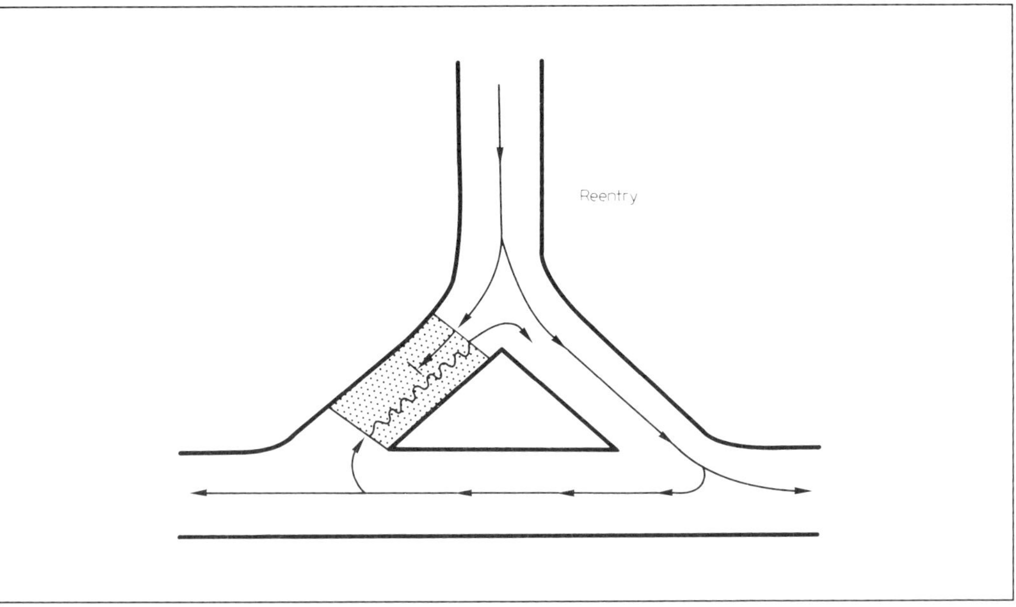
Reentry

2

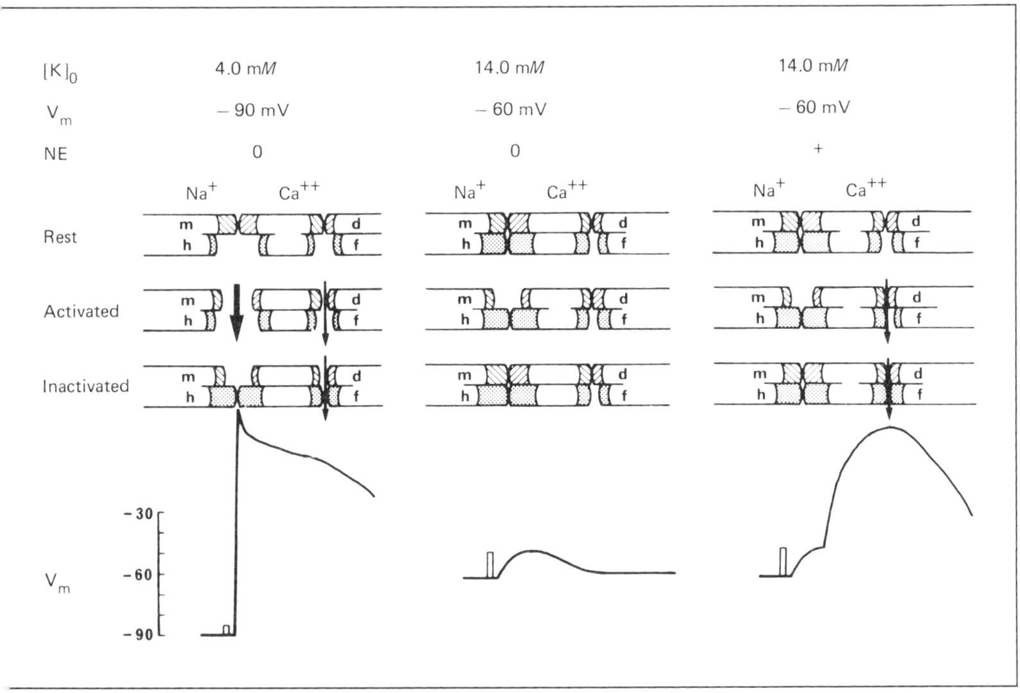
[K]0
4.0 mM
14.0 mM
14.0 mM
Vm
– 90 mV
– 60 mV
– 60 mV
NE
0
0
+
Na+
Ca++
Rest
Activated
Inactivated
m
h
d
f
Vm
-30
-60
-90

3

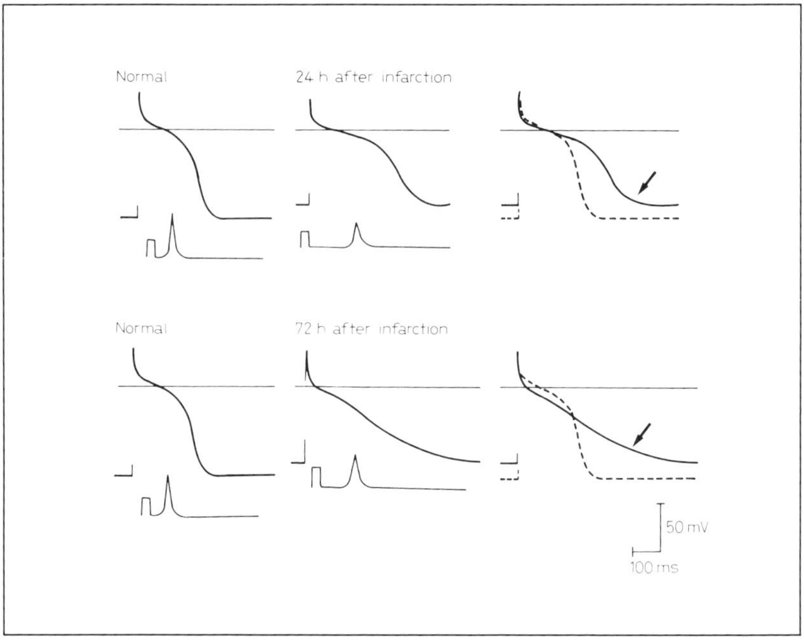

Fig. 4. Comparison of subendocardial Purkinje fiber action potentials 24 and 72 h after experimental myocardial infarction in the dog [from ref. 16, with permission].

decrease in resting membrane potential (fig. 3) closes the fast sodium channels, but not the slow calcium ones. Thus, calcium influx is not prevented, and when it is potentiated by catecholamines or by sympathetic activity, a slow propagating potential develops [16]. Once the periischemic area recovers its excitability, this slow potential can activate it and induce dangerous arrhythmias through reentrant excitability. Ventricular arrhythmias that develop during the first few minutes after a coronary artery of the dog is occluded experimentally are also due to reentrant excitation [6]. This same mechanism is often responsible for the ventricular arrhythmias that occur in man soon after an anterior myocardial infarction [13].

Arrhythmias that develop more than 24 h after experimental infarction in the dog [6] and those seen several hours after myocardial infarction in man [13] appear to be caused primarily by increased automaticity. For example, the action potential of Purkinje cells lengthens progressively in the dog as the time after coronary occlusion increases. Consequently, after depolarization extends further and further into the diastolic period, making automatic reexcitation easier (fig. 4) [16]. Thus, the roles of reentrant excitation and increased automaticity are not always readily distinguishable. Furthermore, evidence has shown that adrenergic hyperactivity may enhance automaticity.

Therapeutic Implications

Distinctions between exertional angina and angina at rest and between reentrant arrhythmias and arrhythmias due to increased automaticity have important therapeutic implications that influence the strategy of intervention. The contribution of cardiac sympathetic activity to some of these disturbances represents the pathophysiologic basis for the use of beta-blockers in angina and arrhythmias.

References

1 Cahine, R.A.: Unstable angina. The problem of definition. Br. Heart J. *37:* 1246–1249 (1975).

2 Chierchia, S.; Brunelli, C.; Simonetti, I.; Lannari, M.; Maseri, A.: Sequence of events in angina at rest: primary reduction in coronary flow. Circulation *61:* 759–768 (1980).

3 Fowler, N.O.: Preinfarction angina. Circulation *44:* 755–758 (1971).

4 Guazzi, M.; Polese, A.; Fiorentini, C.; Macrini, F.; Bartorelli, C.: Left ventricular performance and related haemodynamic changes in Prinzmetal's variant angina pectoris. Br. Heart J. *33:* 84–94 (1971).

5 Heng, M.K.; Norris, R.M.; Singh, B.N.; Partridge, J.B.: Prognosis in unstable angina. Br. Heart J. *38:* 921–925 (1976).

6 Hoffman, B.F.: Role of the sympathetic nervous system in arrhythmias occurring after coronary artery occlusion and myocardial infarction; in Schwartz, Brown, Malliani, Zanchetti, Neural mechanisms in cardiac arrhythmias, pp. 155–166 (Raven Press, New York 1978).

7 Malliani, A.; Lombardi, F.: Neural reflexes associated with myocardial ischemia; in Schwartz, Brown, Malliani, Zanchetti, Neural mechanisms in cardiac arrhythmias, pp. 209–219 (Raven Press, New York 1978).

8 Malliani, A.; Schwartz, P.J.; Zanchetti, A.: A sympathetic reflex elicited by experimental coronary occlusion. Am. J. Physiol. *217:* 703–709 (1969).

9 Malliani, A.; Schwartz, P.J.; Zanchetti, A.: Neural mechanisms in life-threatening arrhythmias. Am. Heart J. *100:* 705–715 (1980).

10 Maseri, A.: Pathogenetic mechanisms of angina pectoris: expanding views. Br. Heart J. *43:* 648–660 (1980).

11 Maseri, A.; L'Abbate, A.; Pesola, A.; Ballestra, A.M.; Marzilli, M.; Maltinti, G.; Serveri, S.; De Nes, D.M.; Parodi, O.; Biagini, A.: Coronary vasospasm in angina pectoris. Lancet *i:* 713–717 (1977).

12 National Heart, Lung and Blood Institute: Report on international activities. October 1, 1980 – September 30, 1981 (Washington 1982).

13 Pantridge, J.P.: Emergency treatment of cardiac arrhythmias in myocardial infarction; in Scott, Julian, Lidocaine in the treatment of ventricular arrhythmias, pp. 77–81 (Livingstone, Edinburgh 1971).

14 Pantridge, J.F.: Autonomic disturbance at the onset of acute myocardial infarction; in Schwartz, Brown, Malliani, Zanchetti, Neural mechanisms in cardiac arrhythmias, pp. 7–17 (Raven Press, New York 1978).

15 Stern, S.; Tzivoni, D.: Early detection of silent ischemic heart disease by 24-hour electrocardiographic monitoring of active subjects. Br. Heart J. *36:* 481–486 (1976).

16 Wit, A.L.; Bigger, J.T.: Possible electrophysiological mechanisms for lethal arrhythmias accompanying myocardial ischemia and infarction. Circulation *51–52:* suppl. 3, pp. 96–115 (1975).

Alberto Zanchetti, Center for Clinical Physiology and Hypertension,
University of Milan, I-20122 Milan (Italy)

Stress and Psychosomatic Disorders

Stevo Julius

Ann Arbor, Mich., USA

Introduction

Whereas such phrases as 'I love my sweetheart' and 'I am heartbroken' reflect the popular notion that emotions and cardiovascular responses are associated, the scientific analysis of this relationship is less than straightforward. *Cannon* [2] viewed the association of the somatovisceral and emotional response to external stimuli as useful and subserving the need for self-protection. Thereafter, it was indeed established that autonomic responses to 'danger' are appropriate as they mobilize the organism to respond with 'fight or flight'. Areas in the brain were defined from which one could elicit a 'defense reaction' [9]. The defense reaction is characterized by an increased cardiac output, blood pressure, and by considerable vasodilation in the muscles – an ideal constellation to enhance motor responses. However, *Zanchetti* et al. [25] were the first to point out the plasticity of the response. As the experience sets in by repetition of the stimuli, the cat responds to an external stimulus with a more specific cardiovascular adaptation; vasodilation may be replaced by vasoconstriction, and the motor pattern may change. This is an important observation as it documents that an individual's experience will largely determine the visceral and motor aspects of the emotional response.

If relatively simple experimental conditions can induce such a plasticity of response in animals, the variety of responses in humans must be bewildering. It is testimony to the elegance of thought and discipline of mind that psychologists have attempted to categorize human responses to stressful stimuli. The discussion evolves around the basic issue – whether autonomic responses are content and situation specific or specific to an individual. Does 'fear' elicit one and 'anger' another stereotype autonomic response? Is there a reproducible 'withdrawal-conversation' versus 'activation-challenge' pattern of autonomic responses? Or does each individual develop his own coping style and his own set of autonomic responses? Psychologists continue to elucidate these issues, but the consensus seems to become more remote as, while striving for precision, each school of thought develops its own nomenclature. Consequently, a common sense summary of our understanding of psychosomatic complexities is in order:

(1) In contemporary society, direct danger is infrequent, and the simple 'fight or flight' reaction is socially unacceptable. Other responses are substituted for these elementary reactions.

(2) Modern stressors are predominantly various demands to perform and achieve. The stress depends on the individual's capacity to react.

(3) The individual's experience is an important determinant of the response: a habitual 'style' develops. The major components of an individual's response are appraisal of the outside stimulus, assessment of one's capacity to respond, and motivation to respond.

(4) Although the outside stimuli are not recognized as a direct threat, they nevertheless cause autonomic responses. These responses need not be hemodynamically stereotypic, but they always involve sympathetic cardiovascular activation.

(5) This autonomic activation, if excessive or inappropriate, may cause cardiovascular disease.

With this background in mind, a short review of the evidence on stress and cardiovascular diseases is in order.

Coronary Heart Disease, Arrhythmias

In 1971, *Jenkins* [12] reviewed a large body of literature on the association between psychosocial factors and coronary heart disease. The interaction is rather complex, since psychosocial factors may influence coronary heart disease indirectly through smoking, overweight, and sodium intake. Older studies were frequently retrospective and had no appropriate control groups, but the results were nevertheless rather informative. *Kits Van Heijningen and Treurniet* [17] reported in 1966 that in many of their patients myocardial infarction was frequently preceded by a loss of prestige, rejection by a loved person, or a setback at work. In the study by *Bruhn* et al. [1]

the emotional factors were associated with coronary deaths. They found a preponderance of long-term life struggles with adversities in the histories of people dying from myocardial infarction. Bereavement appears to be another factor that can provoke myocardial infarction. *Parkes* et al. [22] reported in 1969 a follow-up of 4,486 widowers. During the first 6 months of bereavement, widowers had a 40% excess of deaths over the age-adjusted death rates in the general population. 50% of these excessive deaths were from cardiac causes.

A newer retrospective study of psychosocial risk leading to first myocardial infarction was reported by *Siegrist* et al. [24]. They analyzed 380 surviving men aged 30–55 years. A control group of 190 males of similar job and socioeconomic status was also analyzed. The control group was reasonably well matched in regard to smoking, physical activity, overweight, and hypertension. The focus of the study was on socioeconomic aspects. They analyzed 'strain from life' events 2 years prior to enrollment in the study and found a 4.3:1 ratio of 'high strain' in patients with myocardial infarction versus control subjects. A somewhat better control for traditional risk factors has been presented by *Orth-Gomer* [21]. The study is retrospective, but it matches patients who experienced myocardial infarction with subjects who had similar coronary risk factors (blood pressure, cholesterol, weight, smoking, and alcohol intake). The amount of stress was assessed by a special psychosocial interview. Patients with myocardial infarction had a 6.3:1 ratio of stress-positive interviews compared to patients with equal coronary risk factors. The confounding problem in this study is that the experience of a prior myocardial infarction may sensitize patients to report stressful events.

There is also good evidence that psychosomatic factors influence cardiac arrhythmias. Research into the relationship between cardiac arrhythmia (or sudden death) is difficult due to the sporadic nature of the event. *Lown* [18], however, reviewed the evidence and launched a systematic effort to document the relationship. In 19 patients with frequent ventricular arrhythmia, central sympathetic activation by mental arithmetics, reading from colored cards, and by recounting emotional events increased the frequency of ventricular arrhythmias. Activation of peripheral reflexes by tilt, Valsalva maneuver, and pressure on carotid sinuses failed to alter the frequency of ventricular beats [19]. Apparently arrhythmias cannot be induced by simple reflex activation. Only a complex integrated change in autonomic discharge, such as one encounters with emotions, leads to ventricular arrhythmias. In a later study, *Reich* et al. [23] reported on 117 patients with malignant ventricular arrhythmias. In these patients, in addition to signs of electrical instability of the myocardium, they found a background of 'intense psychological state burdening daily life'. In 21 of these individuals a psychological trigger closely preceded the deranged rhythm.

The overall evidence reviewed in this section suggests that psychosocial factors may be related to the provocation of myocardial infarction and cardiac arrhythmias. The possible relationship of behavioral factors and the development of coronary heart disease will be discussed in the chapter on type A behavior.

Hypertension

A myocardial infarction is a well-defined point, and a stressful event preceding it may be identified easily. The issue is much more complex, with the slowly developing disease of hypertension. Of necessity, the methodology used to document the role of psychosomatic factors in hypertension will be different from those in myocardial infarction. There is tantalizing evidence in the literature that there may be a relationship between psychosocial factors and hypertension; hypertension is (1) more frequent in urban centers than in villages, (2) more prevalent among US blacks who experience more social stress, and (3) entirely absent in some primitive populations. It is impossible, however, to discern whether social stress is an important factor in generating these differences. It is equally possible that increased weight and higher sodium and alcohol intake account for the differences. A superb effort to discern these factors in a natural setting in the city of Detroit was made by *Harburg* et al. [7]. These careful studies indicate that psychosocial stress may be operative in American black hypertensives, but genetic factors are equally important.

Since massive sociopsychological studies in hypertension are difficult, efforts have been made to determine whether hypertensive individuals are (1) more prone to exaggerated responses to psychological stimuli, (2) whether there is evidence for increased sympathetic overactivity in hypertension, and (3) whether the personality characteristics of hypertensive individuals suggest that they may be stress prone.

The best case of psychosomatic influence in hypertension can be made in patients with borderline and mild hypertension. In these cases there is a hyperkinetic state due to increased net autonomic drive to the heart [15] and blood vessels [14]. The catecholamine values in such patients are elevated [3, 6]. These patients respond to mental challenge with an exaggerated blood pressure and increased catecholamine levels [20]. This exaggerated response is also present in normotensive offspring of hypertensive parents [4]. The excessive responsiveness need not be manifest only as a blood pressure increase. *Hollenberg* et al. [10] have shown no increase in blood pressure, but a substantial increase in renal vascular resistance when patients with mild hypertension and offspring of hypertensive parents were exposed to laboratory mental stress. The latter finding is particularly important, since there is no evidence for an overall increased blood pressure variability in the natural setting in such patients [11, 16]. Exaggerated blood pressure responses to mental stimuli may well characterize the laboratory behavior of these individuals, but the mechanism by which such propensity leads to the development of hypertension is not clear. Most assuredly, it is not through repeated 'pressor' episodes, since blood pressure variations outside the laboratory are normal in these patients. It is conceivable that the faster heart rate and blood pressure response are only a marker of some crucial changes in a 'target' vascular bed or of some specific neurohumoral changes. Subtle changes in renal blood flow may lead to sodium retention. Some of these patients show higher levels of plasma renin [6], and the role of this abnormality in the pathogenesis of hypertension requires further elucidation.

Personality testing in patients with mild hypertension, in our hands, gives rather consistent results. Patients are described as submissive and outwardly oriented. These characteristics were evident in students in the USA [8] and in Yugoslavia [13]. Later it was shown that such personality is typical for patients with mild hypertension with biochemical and pharmacologic evidence for sympathetic activity [3]. In this study a questionnaire on anger was utilized for the first time. Patients with mild hypertension were prone to hold 'anger in' and had difficulty expressing it. Clearly, such personality would be more attuned to registering environmental stresses and may well strive further to achieve social goals.

The evidence for psychosomatic factors in hypertension, while good, should not be overrated. Most puzzling is the question of why it is so easy to demonstrate autonomic overactivity in offsprings of hypertensive parents and in the mildest forms of hypertension and why the evidence is so poor in established hypertension. Autonomic overactivity may be the initiating factor for hypertension in some patients. Later on, secondary changes in vascular geometry [5] or in some humoral factors may prevail and be responsible for maintaining the hypertension.

References

1 Bruhn, J.G.; McGrady, K.E.; DuPlessis, A.: Evidence of 'emotional drain' preceding death from myocardial infarction. Psychiat. Dig. *29:* 34–40 (1968).

2 Cannon, W.G.: Bodily changes in pain, hunger, fear and rage (Branford, Boston 1929).

3 Esler, M.; Julius, S.; Sweifler, A.; Randal, O.; Harburg, E.; Gardiner, H.; DeQuattro, V.: Mild high-renin essential hypertension. Neurogenic human hypertension? New Engl. J. Med. *296:* 405–411 (1977).

4 Falkner, B.; Onesti, G.; Angelakos, E.T.; Fernandes, M.; Langman, C.: Cardiovascular response to mental stress in normal adolescents with hypertensive parents. Hemodynamics and mental stress in adolescents. Hypertension *1:* 23–30 (1979).

5 Folkow, B.: Role of vascular factor in hypertension. Contr. Nephrol., vol. 8, pp. 81–94 (Karger, Basel 1977).

6 Goldstein, D.S.: Plasma norepinephrine in essential hypertension. A study of the studies. Hypertension *3:* 48–52 (1981).

7 Harburg, E.; Erfurt, J.C.; Chape, C.; Hauenstein, L.S.; Schull, W.J.; Schork, M.A.: Socio-ecological stress, suppressed hostility, skin color, and black-white male blood pressure: Detroit. Psychosom. Med. *35:* 276–296 (1973).

8 Harburg, E.; Julius, S.; McGinn, N.F.; McLeod, J.; Hoobler, S.W.: Personality traits and behavioral patterns associated with systolic blood pressure levels in college males. J. chron. Dis. *17:* 405–414 (1964).

9 Hess, W.R.: Das Zwischenhirn. Syndrome, Lokalisationen, Funktionen (Schwabe, Basel 1949).

10 Hollenberg, N.K.; Williams, G.H.; Adams, D.F.: Essential hypertension: abnormal renal vascular and endocrine responses to a mild psychological stimulus. Hypertension *3:* 11–17 (1981).

11 Horan, M.J.; Kennedy, H.L.; Padgett, N.E.: Do borderline hypertensive patients have labile blood pressure? Ann. intern. Med. *94:* 466–468 (1981).

12 Jenkins, C.D.: Psychologic and social precursors of coronary disease. New Engl. J. Med. *284:* 244–255 (1971).

13 Julius, S.: The psychophysiology of borderline hypertension; in Weiner, Hofer, Stunkard, Brain, behavior and bodily disease, pp. 293–303 (Raven Press, New York 1981).

14 Julius, S.; Esler, M.: Autonomic nervous cardiovascular regulation in borderline hypertension. Am. J. Cardiol. *36:* 685–696 (1975).

15 Julius, S.; Pascual, A.V.; London, R.: Role of parasympathetic inhibition in the hyperkinetic type of borderline hypertension. Circulation *44:* 413–418 (1971).

16 Julius, S.; Schork, M.A.: Borderline hypertension – a critical review. J. chron. Dis. *23:* 723–754 (1971).

17 Kits Van Heijningen, H.; Treurniet, N.: Psychodynamic factors in acute myocardial infarction. Int. J. Psycho-Analysis *4:* 370–374 (1966).

18 Lown, B.: Mental stress, arrhythmias and sudden death. Am. J. Med. *72:* 177–184 (1982).

19 Lown, B.; DeSilva, R.A.: Roles of psychologic stress and autonomic nervous system changes in provocation of ventricular premature complexes. Am. J. Cardiol. *41:* 979–985 (1978).

20 Nestel, P.J.: Blood pressure and catecholamine excretion after mental stress in labile hypertension. Lancet *i:* 692–694 (1969).
21 Orth-Gomer, K.: Psychosocial stress and CHD when controlling for traditional risk factors; in Siegrist, Myocardial infarction and psychosocial risks, p. 65 (Springer, New York 1981).
22 Parkes, C.M.; Benjamin, B.; Fitzgerald, R.G.: Broken heart: a statistical study of increased mortality among widowers. Br. med. J. *i:* 740–743 (1969).
23 Reich, P.; DeSilva, R.A.; Lown, B.; Murawski, B.J.: Acute psychological disturbance preceding life threatening ventricular arrhythmias. J. Am. med. Ass. *246:* 233–235 (1981).
24 Siegrist, J.; Dittman, K.; Rittner, K.; Weber, I.: Psychosocial risk constellations and first myocardial infarction; in Siegrist, Myocardial infarction and psychosocial risks, p. 41 (Springer, New York 1981).
25 Zanchetti, A.; Baccelli, G.; Mancia, G.: Cardiovascular effects of emotional behavior; in Bartorelli, Zanchetti, Cardiovascular regulation, p. 17 (Istituto di Ricerche Cardiovascolari, Milano 1971).

Stevo Julius, Division of Hypertension, Department of Internal Medicine, University of Michigan Medical School, Ann Arbor, MI 48109 (USA)

Type A Behavior

Stevo Julius
Ann Arbor, Mich., USA

Introduction

As indicated earlier in the general discussion of psychosomatic influences on cardiovascular function, an important factor is the subject's assessment and perception of external stresses. If a challenge in the subject's mind is large and calls for reaction, a cardiovascular response will ensue. People differ in the degree to which they can be challenged and are ready to respond. *Friedman and Rosenman* [8] pointed out already in 1959 that a typical style of behavior is frequently associated with coronary heart disease (CHD). This type A behavior pattern is described as 'an action-emotion complex exhibited by many individuals who are engaged in chronic struggle to obtain unlimited numbers of things from their environment in the shortest period of time, often in spite of other things and persons. This "struggle" is a competitive attempt to do and to achieve more in less and less time' [17]. The goals of such individuals are ever expanding; there is always something new to achieve. Type A individuals are not overly anxious, they, in fact, profess to enjoy the challenge and are confident in their capacity to prevail. The point is made that type A is not a fixed personality, but a behavioral syndrome. Consequently, the behavior will be elicited with proper stimuli, but if left unchallenged, a type A individual may not differ much from one with the opposite, type B, behavior. When challenged, a type A will exhibit a number of traits: aggressiveness, impatience, and, not infrequently, also hostility. Another facet of the provoked behavior is alertness, rapid and emphatic speech, and motoric unrest. Type A individuals frequently have poor insight, particularly in appraising their own capacity to meet challenges. Because of this time urgency that type A persons so characteristically display, various questionnaires are not uniformly successful in uncovering type A traits. *Rosenman and Chesney* [17] prefer using a structured interview to elicit type A behavior. It requires 15 min and ideally is audio- and videotaped for subsequent evaluation.

Trained individuals can then rate the interview which is structured to elicit specific facets of type A behavior. In the analysis, more attention is paid to the individual style of responding than to the content of the interview. If a trained structured interviewer is not available, type A behavior can be assessed by the Jenkins Activity Survey [15]. Whereas this questionnaire shows a relationship to CHD in field studies, the power of prediction is poorer than that of the structured interview [17]. An important facet of type A behavior is hostility which will not be uncovered by the Jenkins Activity Survey questionnaire. The Bortner Rating Scale [2] correlates well with the structured interview, but has not been widely used.

Type A and CHD

The initial observation by *Friedman and Rosenman* [8] and by *Rosenman and Friedman* [18] that type A and CHD are cross-sectionally associated has been amply verified [3, 4, 11, 23]. Cross-sectional studies, however, do not provide the answer about the nature of the relationship. If type A is to be implicated as a pathophysiologic factor, it must precede the development of CHD. Therefore, of more interest are prospective studies of subjects who are free of CHD and display type A behavior. The Western Collaborative Group Study is one example of such a prospective trial [21, 22]; 3,154 employed men, aged 39–59 years, were followed for 8.5 years. Of these subjects, 25% developed ischemic heart disease. Factors that predict the development of CHD in order of magnitude were cholesterol level, behavior pattern, cigarette smoking, and the systolic blood pressure. Multiple logistic analysis was applied to the data. This statistical method allows assessment of the independent contribution of each factor to the coronary risk. The overall incidence of CHD in type A was 2.37 times as frequent as in type B. When statistical adjustment for other risk factors was made, the type A group still had 1.97 times a chance to develop CHD than the type B.

Results of the Western Cooperative Group Study are impressive, but their general applicability is limited by the nature of the population. All subjects were middle-class men. The population in the Framingham Study is more representative. This study of a community in Massachusetts has been the main source of reliable data on cardiovascular risk factors in the United States. In 1965 and in 1967, a questionnaire was given to 750 women and 580 men aged 45–64 and clinically free of CHD [13]. An update of these results, just recently published [12], includes prospective observations of minimum 4 and maximum of 10 years. Among women the incidence of CHD was double in type A compared to their type B counterparts. This incidence was higher among housewives amounting to 2.5 more than in type B. Incidence of CHD in type A working mean was 2.4 more than in the type B. This study found that clinical manifestations of CHD in type A are different. Type A individuals tend to have overt angina pectoris. The Framingham Study investigators have also analyzed the association of type A risk with other risk factors. This is shown in table I. When type A is superimposed on other risk factors, the overall risk is higher. The exceptions are very low systolic blood pressure and frequent cigarette smoking.

Pathophysiologic Correlates of Type A Behavior

Does type A behavior precipitate manifestations of the underlying CHD, or does the A behavior contribute to the development of coronary atherosclerosis? Angiographic studies suggest that type A behavior may well be related to the development and worsening of coronary atherosclerosis [1, 5, 6, 16, 24, 25].

In these clinical studies type A patients tend to have a higher prevalence and more severe coronary atherosclerosis. Clinical studies are frequently plagued by methodological problems particularly in regards to the selection of the material. Nevertheless, it would be frivolous to suggest that type A individuals choose to have angiography, when the disease is advanced. The epidemiologic association is strong and, if anything, suggests that type A individuals experience earlier and more symptoms [12] than do type B.

Since type A behavior is associated also with an excess of coronary deaths as well as with more anginal symptoms, on conceptual grounds one must also accept the possibility that type A behavior precipitates manifestations of already developed CHD.

Little is known about the pathophysiology of the type A behavior pattern, but whatever evidence there is, it delineates a precipitating rather than an etiologic role of type A in the natural history of CHD. A hyperadrenergic state has been associated with type A behavior. Type A individuals show a

Table I. CHD risk according to type A behavior and standard coronary risk factors [from ref. 13]

Standard risk factors	10-year incidence of CHD, %			
	men 45–64 years		women 45–64 years	
	type B (n = 294)	type A (n = 276)	type B (n = 372)	type A (n = 348)
Systolic blood pressure, mm Hg				
<120	10.0	7.5	5.0	6.8
120–159	11.7	18.7	4.7	10.2
≧160	22.0	38.7	8.5	16.9
Diastolic blood pressure, mm Hg				
<95	12.0	15.8	5.1	9.4
≧95	18.2	38.2	8.1	18.4
Serum cholesterol, mg/100 ml				
<220	9.8	12.4	6.0	6.5
220–259	13.1	22.2	3.5	7.5
≧260	19.1	26.9	8.2	19.0
Cigarettes smoked per day				
0	10.5	17.0	5.3	10.1
1–20	14.9	23.2	5.8	10.3
≧21	15.6	16.7	3.4	14.7

higher catecholamine excretion during working hours [10]. Their catecholamine response to specific behavioral challenge is also exaggerated [7]. If these findings reflect the naturally occurring events, an excess of sympathetic drive may be responsible for arrhythmias, angina, and sudden death. Type A subjects respond to environmental challenges with an excessive elevation of serum cholesterol levels [9, 19]. Serum cholesterol levels in the resting state are, however, only minimally elevated [8, 18, 20]. It is not known whether these acute elevations of cholesterol have a pathophysiologically important effect. Finally, hematologic findings in type A are of interest. It has been suggested that subjects with type A behavior pattern have accelerated blood clotting and an increased platelet aggregation [9, 14]. This conceivably could precipitate acute coronary thrombosis.

References

1 Blumenthal, J.A.; Williams, R.B.; Kong, Y.; Schanberg, S.M.; Thompson, L.W.: Type A behavior pattern and coronary atherosclerosis. Circulation *58:* 634–639 (1978).

2 Bortner, R.W.: A short rating scale as a potential measure of pattern A behavior. J. chron. Dis. *22:* 87–91 (1969).

3 Caffrey, B.: Behaviour patterns and personality characteristics related to prevalence rates of CHD in American monks. J. chron. Dis. *22:* 93–103 (1970).

4 Cohen, J.B.; Syme, J.L.; Jenkins, C.D.; Kagan, A.; Zyzanski, S.J.: Cultural context of type A behavior and risk for CHD: a study of Japanese-American males. J. Behav. Med. *2:* 475–484 (1979).

5 Dimsdale, J.E.; Hackett, T.P.; Hutter, A.M.; Block, P.C.; Catanzano, D.M.: Type A personality and extent of coronary atherosclerosis. Am. J. Cardiol. *42:* 583–586 (1978).

6 Frank, K.A.; Heller, S.S.; Kornfeld, D.S.; Sporn, A.A.; Weiss, M.D.: Type A behavior pattern and coronary atherosclerosis. J. Am. med. Ass. *240:* 761–763 (1978).

7 Friedman, M.; Byers, S.O.; Diamant, J.; Rosenman, R.H.: Plasma catecholamine response to coronary-prone subjects (type A) to a specific challenge. Metabolism *24:* 205–210 (1975).

8 Friedman, M.; Rosenman, R.H.: Association of specific overt behavior pattern with blood and cardiovascular findings. J. Am. med. Ass. *169:* 1286–1296 (1959).

9 Friedman, M.; Rosenman, R.H.; Carrol, V.: Changes in the serum cholesterol and blood clotting time in men subjected to cyclic variation of occupational stress. Circulation *17:* 852–855 (1958).

10 Friedman, M.; St. George, S.; Byers, S.O.; Rosenman, R.H.: Excretion of catecholamines, 17-ketosteroids, 17-hydroxycorticoids, and 5-hydroxyindole in men exhibiting a particular behavior pattern (A) associated with high incidence of clinical coronary artery disease. J. clin. Invest. *39:* 758–764 (1960).

11 Haynes, S.G.; Feinleib, M.; Levine, S.; Scoth, N.; Kannel, W.B.: The relationship of psychosocial factors to coronary heart disease in the Framingham Study. II. Prevalence of coronary heart disease. Am. J. Epidem. *107:* 384–402 (1978).

12 Haynes, S.G.; Feinleib, M.; Eaker, E.D.: Type A behavior and the 10 year incidence of coronary heart disease in the Framingham Heart Study; in Rosenman, Psychosomatic risk factors and coronary heart disease: indications for specific preventive therapy (Huber, Bern 1983).

13 Haynes, S.G.; Feinleib, M.; Kannel, W.B.: The relationship of psychosocial factors to coronary heart disease in the Framingham Study. III. Eight-year incidence of coronary heart disease. Am. J. Epidem. *111:* 37–58 (1980).

14 Jenkins, C.D.; Thomas, G.; Olewine, D.; Zyzanski, S.J.; Simpson, M.T.; Hames, C.G.: Blood platelet aggregation and personality traits. J. hum. Stress *1:* 34–46 (1975).

15 Jenkins, C.D.; Rosenman, R.H.; Zyzanski, S.J.: Jenkins Activity Survey (Psychological Corp., New York 1979).

16 Krantz, D.S.; Sanmario, M.I.; Selvester, R.H.; Matthews, K.A.: Psychological correlates of progression of atherosclerosis in men. Psychosom. Med. *41:* 467–475 (1979).

17 Rosenman, R.H.; Chesney, M.A.: Psychological profiles and coronary heart disease; in Kielholz, Siegenthaler, Taggart, Zanchetti, Psychosomatic cardiovascular disorders – when and how to treat? (Huber, Bern 1981).
18 Rosenman, R.H.; Friedman, M.: Association of specific behavior pattern in women with blood and cardiovascular findings. Circulation *24:* 1173–1184 (1961).
19 Rosenman, R.H.; Friedman, M.: Neurogenic factors in pathogenesis of coronary heart disease. Med. Clins N. Am. *58:* 269–279 (1974).
20 Rosenman, R.H.; Friedman, M.: Behavior patterns, blood lipids, and coronary heart disease. J. Am. med. Ass. *184:* 934–938 (1963).
21 Rosenman, R.H.; Friedman, M.; Straus, R.; Wurm, M.; Kositchek, R.; Hahn, W.; Wethessen, N.T.: A predictive study of coronary heart disease. The Western Collaborative Group Study. J. Am. med. Ass. *189:* 15–22 (1964).
22 Rosenman, R.H.; Jenkins, C.D.; Brand, R.J.; Friedman, M.; Straus, R.; Wurm, M.: Coronary heart disease in the Western Collaborative Group Study: a final follow-up experience of 8.5 years. J. Am. med. Ass. *233:* 872–877 (1975).
23 Shekelle, R.B.; Schoenberger, S.A.; Stamler, J.: Correlates of the JAS type A behavior pattern score. J. chron. Dis. *29:* 381–394 (1976).
24 Williams, R.B.; Haney, T.L.; Lee, K.L.; Kong, Y.H.; Blumenthal, J.A.; Whalen, R.E.: Type A behavior, hostility, and coronary atherosclerosis. Psychosom. Med. *42:* 539–549 (1980).
25 Zyzanski, S.J.; Jenkins, C.D.; Ryan, R.J.; Flessas, A.; Everist, M.: Psychological correlates of coronary angiographic findings. Archs intern. Med. *136:* 1234–1237 (1976).

Stevo Julius, Division of Hypertension, Department of Internal Medicine,
University of Michigan Medical School, Ann Arbor, MI 48109 (USA)

II. Strategy of Intervention

Beta-Blockers as First-Line Defense

Alberto Zanchetti
Milan, Italy

Review of Available Beta-Blockers

History

The development of chemical compounds capable of selectively antagonizing some of the actions of sympathetic stimulation, leaving others unaffected, was influenced by *Ahlquist* [1]. He developed the concept that the most important link in the adrenergic neuroeffector transmission chain was represented by adrenoceptors and proposed that there are two types: alpha-receptors, which in the cardiovascular system mediate vasoconstriction, and beta-receptors which mediate vasodilation and myocardial stimulation. As often occurs with discoveries published ahead of their time, *Ahlquist's* concept was largely ignored by the scientific community. However, *Powell and Slater* [11] used *Ahlquist's* hypothesis to classify the pharmacologic properties of dichloroisoproterenol, and subsequently *Black* et al. [3] and *Black and Stephenson* [4] developed pronethalol and propranolol, the first clinically useful beta-receptor blockers [2, 7].

Beta-Blockade in Man

A host of compounds with beta-adrenergic blocking activity are currently available. Those most widely used clinically are listed in table I. The one property they have in common is their ability to block beta-adrenergic receptors. In man this property is generally determined by measuring the heart rate responses to either increasing doses of the beta-adrenergic agonist isoproterenol or to increasing degrees of exercise, both before and after the intravenous or oral administration of a beta-blocker. Thus, stimulus-response curves can be described which characterize the response of cardiac receptors. These curves are shifted to the right by compounds with beta-receptor antagonism.

Cardioselectivity

A comparison of the various beta-blockers has shown that they may possess additional properties, some of which may be clinically relevant. The term cardioselectivity indicates that some compounds selectively bind to cardiac beta-receptors in preference to beta-receptors located in bronchi and blood vessels [8]. This observation has led to the subclassification of beta-receptors as beta-1 and beta-2, with cardioselective blockers acting preferentially as beta-1-receptors.

Selectivity, however, is a relative phenomenon. It can usually be seen at rather small dose levels of the selective compound, but often is lost when large doses are given. The main clinical advantage of a beta-1 or cardioselective blocker is that it may be better tolerated by patients with asthma and chronic bronchitis. Despite this advantage, however, beta-1-selective blockers should be used with caution in patients with respiratory obstructive disease. Atenolol, metoprolol and betaxolol are beta-1- or cardioselective blockers (table I). Practolol, the first cardioselective beta-blocker described, has been withdrawn from clinical use because of toxic side effects that fortunately have not been observed with other beta-blockers.

Table I. Properties of various beta-adrenoreceptor-blocking compounds

Compound	Cardio-selectivity	ISA	Membrane-stabilizing activity	Metabolism and excretion
Propranolol	0	0	++	hepatic
Practolol	+	++	+	renal
Oxprenolol	0	++	+	hepatic
Timolol	0	0	0	hepatic, renal
Pindolol	0	+++	+	hepatic, renal
Metoprolol	+	0	0	hepatic
Atenolol	+	0	0	renal
Alprenolol	0	++	+	hepatic
Acebutolol	0[a]	+	0	renal, hepatic
Sotalol	0	0	0	renal
Nadolol	0	0	0	renal

[a] Not selective in humans [17].

0 indicates lack of a given activity; one or more + indicate increasing degrees of a given activity.

Intrinsic Sympathomimetic Activity (ISA)

ISA or partial agonism is a property shared by some beta-blockers which not only block but also partially stimulate the beta-receptors. This property was particularly marked with dichloroisoproterenol, a compound that caused tachycardia and which, therefore, could not be used therapeutically. A minor degree of ISA can be present and may even offer an advantage in some of the clinically useful beta-blockers. It is most marked with pindolol and is also present to a less marked but nevertheless significant degree in oxprenolol and alprenolol and to a lesser degree in acebutolol.

Beta-blockers with ISA usually induce less bradycardia at rest, although they reduce exercise-induced tachycardia, as do compounds devoid of agonist activity [5]. Utilizing the ISA to stabilize cardiac sympathetic excitation without influencing heart rate at rest too markedly, i.e., when the drug's agonism may predominate over its antagonism, but abolishing excessive endogenous stimulation during stress or exercise, i.e., when antagonism predominates over agonism, is a promising clinical concept of treatment of cardiac disease that should be investigated further [12].

Membrane-Stabilizing Activity

Another property of beta-blockers such as propranolol, oxprenolol, pindolol, and others is their membrane-stabilizing activity. These drugs reduce the rate of rise and the overshoot of the myocardial action potential [16]; electrophysiologic changes similar to those caused by quinidine, hence the term quinidine-like action. It is, however, important to state that the presence or absence of membrane-stabilizing activity is of little significance in the clinical use of beta-blockers for hypertension.

Pharmacokinetics of Beta-Blockers

The pharmacokinetics of various beta-blockers are different, and this is clinically relevant. Administered orally, most beta-blockers are well absorbed across the intestinal mucosa and then subject to first-pass metabolism in the liver. The extent of this first-pass phenomenon is proportional to the lipophilicity of the compound and also shows marked interindividual variability. More lipophilic compounds, such as propranolol, oxprenolol, and alprenolol, undergo more conspicuous hepatic extraction, and their bioavailability is often poor and variable. On the other hand, more hydrophilic compounds, although less completely absorbed, are only slightly subject to hepatic metabolism and are largely excreted through the kidney. Their bioavailability is less variable. Hydrophilic beta-blockers also have a long half-life; their pharmacologic and therapeutic actions are more prolonged, particularly those of atenolol, nadolol, sotalol, and betaxolol.

The duration of action of many beta-blockers has been found to be longer than that which could be predicted from plasma half-life alone. Even beta-blockers with relatively short half-lives have been shown to be effective over a 24-hour period, when they are given in no more than two daily doses. Furthermore, slow-release preparations are available which make it possible to administer both propranolol and oxprenolol in single daily doses, as can be done with naturally long-acting beta-blockers.

Adverse Effects and Contraindications

Absolute contraindications to the clinical use of beta-blockers are: (1) heart failure and all conditions in which cardiac reserve is thought to be markedly reduced and to be critically maintained by cardiac sympathetic activity; (2) airway-obstructive diseases, because bronchodilatation is maintained through beta-2-mediated sympathetic activity, and (3) atrioventricular conduction disturbances with the possible exception of a first-degree atrioventricular block. Removal of sympathetic facilitation of atrioventricular conduction can markedly worsen the clinical condition. Relative contraindications are marked resting bradycardia, insulin-dependent diabetes mellitus (beta-blockers can interfere with catecholamine-mediated glucose release and, therefore, may worsen and mask insulin-induced hypoglycemia), and peripheral arterial disease (claudication is often aggravated by a reduction in cardiac output and the blockage of beta-2-mediated vasodilation). Minor adverse effects are represented by fatigue – probably related to decreased cardiac output –, cold hands and feet, and sometimes Raynaud's phenomenon – related to the same mechanisms aggravating claudication –, sleep disturbances, and nightmares. Sleep disturbances seem to be more marked with lipophilic drugs that move more freely across the blood-brain barrier. Toxic effects such as eye lesions and retroperitoneal fibrosis have only been noted after practolol which has been withdrawn from clinical use.

Hemodynamic Changes Caused by Beta-Blockers

Blood Pressure, Cardiac Output, and Total Vascular Resistance. All beta-blockers, either after intravenous or oral administration, reduce cardiac output both at rest and during exercise. In normotensive individuals, little or no simultaneous reduction in blood pressure occurs. However, when beta-blockers are administered to hypertensive patients, blood pressure is usually reduced. The main problem, hemodynamically, is whether or not there is also a parallel reduction in the elevated vascular resistance which is characteristically elevated in hypertension.

One of the first studies of propranolol [15] showed that its intravenous administration markedly reduced cardiac output without affecting blood pressure, thus increasing total vascular resistance. After oral administration, the antihypertensive effect of propranolol was accompanied by a gradual return of peripheral vascular resistance to pretreatment or to slightly lower values. More recently, however, *Lund-Johansen* [9] reported that even after 2 years of treatment with the beta-1-selective blocker atenolol, the persistent decrease in blood pressure was accompanied by a reduced cardiac output and an increased vascular resistance. Thus, it appears that beta-1-selectivity, although having the potential advantage of not interfering with the vasodilating beta-2-receptors, cannot prevent the further rise in an already elevated vascular resistance associated with the antihypertensive effect of a beta-blocker.

Whether ISA reduces the depressing effect on cardiac output, thereby preventing the rise in vascular resistance, has been questioned. In a recent survey of the literature on the acute and long-term hemodynamic effects of ten different beta-blockers, *Man In't Veld and Schalekamp* [10] have found that the degree of cardiac output depression induced by the various beta-blockers is inversely correlated with their ISA, both in acute and in long-term studies. Vascular resistance, in long-term studies, was higher during treatment with a beta-blocker devoid of ISA than with one containing ISA.

Muscle Blood Flow and Exercise Performance. Several recent studies have shown that a beta-blocker with ISA, such as oxprenolol, induces a smaller reduction in both resting and muscle blood flow after exercise than nonselective or cardioselective beta-blockers without ISA [13, 14]. The relatively normal muscle blood flow and cardiac output maintained by ISA-containing beta-blockers might well explain the improved exercise performance of patients treated with oxprenolol compared with those receiving propranolol [6].

References

1 Ahlquist, R.P.: A study of the adrenotropic receptors. Am. J. Physiol. *153:* 586–600 (1948).

2 Alleyne, G.A.O.; Dickinson, C.J.; Dornhorst, A.C.; Fulton, R.M.; Green, K.G.; Hall, I.D.; Horst, P.; Laurence, D.R.; Pilkington, T.; Prichard, B.N.C.; Robinson, B.;

Rosenheim, M.L.: Effect of pronethalol in angina pectoris. Br. med. J. *ii:* 1226–1229 (1963).
3 Black, J.W.; Duncan, W.A.M.; Shanks, R.G.: Comparison of some properties of pronethalol and propranolol. Br. J. Pharmacol. *25:* 577–591 (1965).
4 Black, J.W.; Stephenson, J.S.: Pharmacology of a new adrenergic beta-receptor blocking compound (nethalide). Lancet *ii:* 311–314 (1962).
5 Dresel, P.E.: Blockade of some cardiac actions of adrenaline by dichloroisoprenaline. Can. J. Biochem. Physiol. *38:* 375–381 (1960).
6 Franciosa, J.A.; Johnson, S.M.; Tobian, J.L.: Exercise performance in mildly hypertensive patients. Impairment by propranolol but not oxprenolol. Chest *78:* 291–299 (1980).
7 Hamer, J.; Grandjean, T.; Melendez, L.; Sowton, G.E.: Effect of propranolol (Inderal) in angina pectoris: preliminary report. Br. med. J. *ii:* 720–723 (1964).
8 Lands, A.M.; Luduena, F.P.; Buzzo, H.J.: Differentiation of receptors responsive to isoproterenol. Life Sci. *6:* 2241–2249 (1967).
9 Lund-Johansen, P.: Hemodynamic consequences of long-term beta-blocker therapy: a 5-year follow-up study of atenolol. J. cardiovasc. Pharmacol. *1:* 487–495 (1979).
10 Man In't Veld, A.J.; Schalekamp, M.A.D.H.: How intrinsic sympathomimetic activity modulates the haemodynamic responses to β-adrenoreceptor antagonists. A clue to the nature of their antihypertensive mechanism. Br. J. clin. Pharmacol. *13:* 245S–257S (1982).
11 Powell, C.E.; Slater, I.H.: Blocking of inhibitory adrenergic receptors by a dichloroanalog of isoproterenol. J. Pharmac. exp. Ther. *122:* 480–488 (1958).
12 Reale, A.; Motolese, M.: Partial agonist activity of beta-adrenergic blocking agents and cardiac performance: a review. Eur. Heart J. *2:* 245–251 (1981).
13 Smith, R.S.; Warren, D.J.: Effect of acute oral beta-adrenergic blockade on muscle blood flow in man. Cardiovasc. Res. *16:* 205–208 (1982).
14 Tarazi, R.C.; Dustan, H.P.: Beta-adrenergic blockade in hypertension. Practical and theoretical implications of long-term hemodynamic variations. Am. J. Cardiol. *29:* 633–640 (1972).
15 Vandenburg, M.J.; Conlon, C.; Ledingham, J.M.: A comparison of the effects of propranolol and oxprenolol on forearm blood flow and skin temperature. Br. J. clin. Pharmacol. *11:* 485–490 (1981).
16 Vaughan Williams, E.M.: The mode of action of beta-receptor antagonists on cardiac muscle. Am. J. Cardiol. *18:* 399–405 (1966).
17 Whitsett, L.: Comparison of the $beta_1$ and $beta_2$ adrenoceptor blocking properties of acebutolol and propranolol. Chest *82:* 668 (1982).

Alberto Zanchetti, Center for Clinical Physiology and Hypertension,
University of Milan, I–20122 Milan (Italy)

Hypertension

Alberto Zanchetti
Milan, Italy

Effectiveness of Beta-Blockers

All beta-blockers, independent of their other pharmacodynamic properties or characteristics, lower the blood pressure of hypertensive patients. Most experts have found that beta-blockers are effective in about 50% of patients with mild or moderate essential hypertension. When administered in association with diuretics or vasodilators, they exert a useful antihypertensive effect in an even higher percentage of hypertensive patients, including those with severe hypertension. Blood pressure has also been lowered to a useful degree in patients with renovascular hypertension treated with beta-blockers alone or in combination with a diuretic, vasodilator, or both. Figure 1, from the recommendations of the WHO expert committee [14], shows that the beta-blockers are now the preferred agents for the treatment of hypertension. The reasons that beta-blockers are, along with diuretics, considered as first-choice treatment are: (1) beta-blockers lower blood pressure both in the supine and in the upright position without interfering with orthostatic control of blood pressure; (2) systolic and diastolic values are both lowered; (3) the antihypertensive effectiveness of the beta-blockers is maintained without attenuation for years, and (4) the incidence and severity of adverse effects are quite limited, provided that contraindications are carefully avoided.

At this point it should be stressed that newer prospective clinical trials favor the use of drugs to treat mild hypertension. This is due in part to the

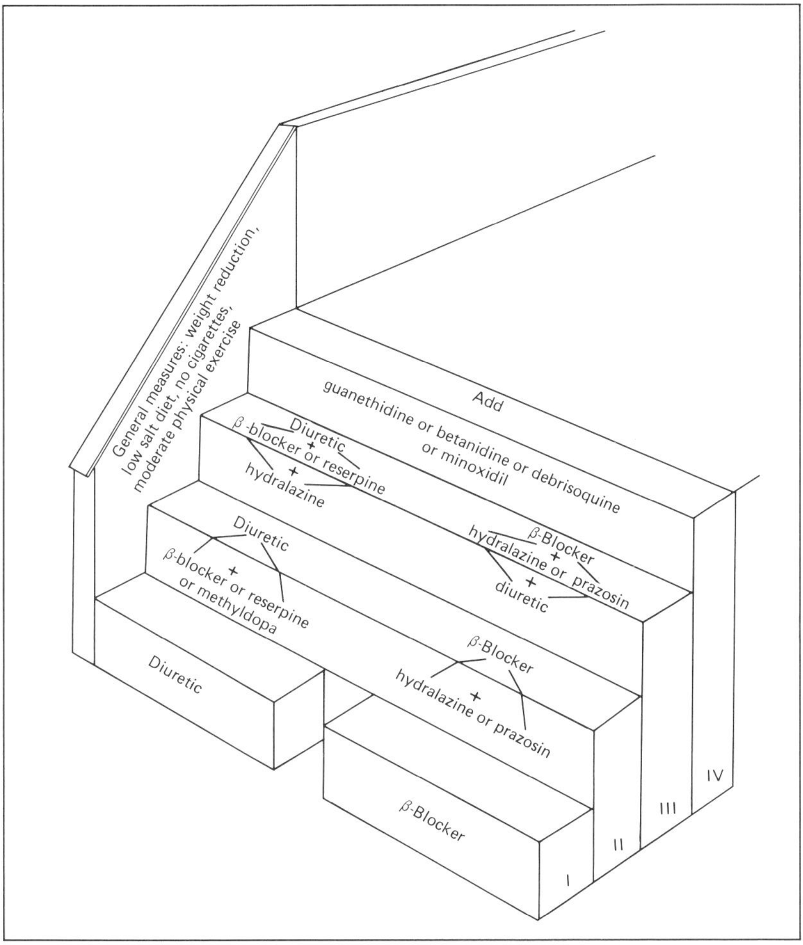

Fig. 1. Stepped care program for the management of hypertensive patients [from ref. 14].

availability of well-tolerated beta-blockers. Some of these drugs, especially propranolol and oxprenolol, have been used to treat hypertension for more than 15 years without causing major problems and with increasingly evident success. Furthermore, the cardioprotective action of the beta-blockers might well reduce the incidence of coronary complications in hypertensive patients once their use becomes widespread. In those prospective studies in which beta-blockers were either not used or were used only sparingly for antihypertensive therapy, cerebrovascular events were clearly reduced but the incidence of coronary disease had not improved [4, 9, 16]. The only study in which coronary mortality and morbidity were reduced by antihypertensive medication was carried out in Sweden where beta-blockers are widely used [2]. Currently underway is a large international prospective study in hypertension [7] which is investigating the suggestion that beta-blockers – in this case slow-release oxprenolol – may help extend the benefits of antihypertensive therapy to the prevention of coronary disease.

Mechanisms of the Antihypertensive Effect of Beta-Blockers

The antihypertensive effect of beta-blockers was discovered serendipitously, when *Prichard* [11] found that these drugs reduced the blood pressure of patients treated for angina. This observation was totally unexpected; there was no pathophysiologic reason to assume that beta-blockers will have antihypertensive properties. After 20 years, and despite several ingenious theories, the mechanism of this effect is still largely unknown.

The first hypothesis suggested that the blood pressure lowering effect of the beta-blockers resulted from a fall in cardiac output. However, as stated in the previous chapter, beta-blockers with intrinsic sympathomimetic activity cause little or no reduction in cardiac output, although they can definitely lower blood pressure. The author has also shown that the cardiac effect of a beta-blocker like propranolol generally occurs at a lower dose and plasma concentration than those required for hypotensive activity [15]. The possibility that beta-blockers might reset baroreflexes, thus reducing blood pressure, has not been substantiated by recent experiments [6].

Inhibition of the release of renin from juxtaglomerular cells, thus suppressing plasma renin activity, has been the most popular hypothesis concerning the antihypertensive effect of the beta-blockers [3]. This theory implies that plasma renin levels could identify – to a clinically useful degree – patients whose blood pressure would respond to the beta-blockers, i.e., patients with high or normal plasma renin concentrations. Low renin concentrations in plasma were reportedly associated with unresponsiveness to beta-blockers but sensitivity to diuretics.

The renin theory has been widely criticized, but most investigators now agree that renin suppression plays a minor role in the antihypertensive effect of beta-blockers [16]. With propranolol, renin suppression occurs at much lower plasma levels of the drug than are required to lower blood pressure. Furthermore, beta-blockers with intrinsic sympathomimetic activity lower blood pressure without reducing plasma renin activity. However, in patients with very high plasma renin levels or those in whom plasma renin is markedly stimulated by concurrent diuretic or vasodilator therapy, the blood pressure lowering effect of the beta-blockers is partly mediated through suppression of elevated plasma renin.

Another series of interpretations directly involve the sympathetic control of circulation. The blocking effects of propranolol on the blood pressure rise induced in animals by the intracisternal injection of isoproterenol has led to the hypothesis that beta-adrenergic receptor mechanisms are involved in the central control of blood pressure and that beta-blockers may exert their antihypertensive effects by interfering with these mechanisms [4, 8]. In fact, many beta-blockers produce central nervous system effects, such as sleep disturbances and nightmares. The more hydrophilic compounds, e.g., atenolol, however, cross the blood-brain barrier only to a very slight extent. Nevertheless, these compounds exert a clear-cut antihypertensive effect. Unless areas of the brain critical for lowering blood pressure are those in which the blood-brain barrier is naturally low, it is unlikely that the antihypertensive effect of beta-blockers results from an action on central beta-receptors.

Another hypothesis, which also involves the sympathetic nervous system, was revived recently to explain the effect of beta-blockers on blood pressure. There is evidence that adrenaline can enhance noradrenergic transmission at the sympathetic postganglionic ending by acting on prejunctional beta-adrenergic receptors [1]. This facilitory influence could be exerted both by circulating and by adrenaline stored in neuronal transmitters and subsequently released as a cotransmitter. In support of this hypothesis, *Tung* et al. [12] recently showed that the prolonged intraperitoneal infusion of minute amounts of adrenaline can slowly induce hypertension in rats. Beta-blockers could interfere with this positive feedback mechanism, potentiating the adrenergic control of circulation, so that blood pressure is lowered. However, there is no direct experimental support for this action by the beta-blockers, and to the extent to which plasma noradrenaline is considered an index of sympathetic activity, no decrease in plasma noradrenaline has been observed, when blood pressure is also lowered by the beta-blockers. Therefore, the mechanism of the antihypertensive effect of these compounds is still unknown.

Role of Intrinsic Sympathomimetic Activity in the Antihypertensive Action of Beta-Blockers

As stated earlier, intrinsic sympathomimetic activity (or partial agonist activity) is not indispensable to the antihypertensive effectiveness of beta-blockers. In principle, excessive beta-agonism might overcome the beta-antagonism in which the antihypertensive properties reside. This does not apply to compounds with moderate partial agonism, such as oxprenolol and pindolol, the antihypertensive activity of which are well established. On the other hand, a moderate degree of partial agonism may provide some advantage; a lesser degree of cardiac depression would play a favorable role in only a limited number of hypertensive patients, especially those with important cardiac involvement and possibly in elderly subjects [16].

Intrinsic sympathomimetic activity, however, has been shown to be associated with a reduction, rather than an increase, in total vascular resistance [10]. Therefore, the hemodynamic pattern of hypertension is normalized more appropriately by intrinsic sympathomimetic activity beta-blockers than by those without intrinsic sympathomimetic activity which lower blood pressure but raise vascular resistance. Furthermore, the better exercise tolerance described in patients receiving beta-blockers with intrinsic sympathomimetic activity suggest that these drugs might help to maintain compliance [5] with therapy in a condition such as arterial hypertension where it is of fundamental importance.

References

1 Adler-Grashinski, E.; Langer, S.Z.: Possible role of beta-adrenoceptor in the regulation of noradrenaline release by nerve stimulation through a positive feedback mechanism. Br. J. Pharmacol. *53:* 43–50 (1975).

2 Berglund, G.; Wilhelmen, L.; Sannerstedt, R.; Hansson, L.; Andersson, O.; Solvertsson, R.; Wedel, H.; Wirkstrand, J.: Coronary heart disease after treatment of hypertension. Lancet *i:* 1–5 (1978).

3 Bühler, F.R.; Laragh, J.H.; Baer, L.; Vaughan, E.D., Jr.; Brunner, H.R.: Propranolol inhibition of renin secretion. A specific approach to diagnosis and treatment of renin-dependent hypertensive diseases. New Engl. J. Med. *287:* 1209–1214 (1972).

4 Day, M.D.; Peters, A.S.; Roach, A.G.: β-Adrenergic receptor blocking agents: evidence for the brain as a site for their cardiovascular effects; in Onesti, Fernandes, Kim, Regulation of blood pressure by the central nervous system, pp. 303–315 (Grune & Stratton, New York 1976).

5 Franciosa, J.A.; Johnson, S.M.; Tobian, J.L.: Exercise performance in mildly hypertensive patients. Impairment by propranolol but not oxprenolol. Chest *78:* 291–299 (1980).

6 Grassi, G.; Gavazzi, C.; Parati, G.; Pomidossi, G.; Ramirez, A.; Bertinieri, G.; Mancia, G.: Baroreceptor control of the cardiovascular system during administration of beta-adrenergic blocking drugs in man. Proc. 1st Eur. Meet. on Hypertension. J. Hypertension (in press, 1983).

7 IPPPSH Group: International prospective primary prevention study in hypertension (IPPPSH) – objectives, design and preliminary data review; in Burley, Birdwood, The clinical impact of beta-adrenoceptor blockade, pp. 193–203 (Ciba Laboratories, Horsham 1980).

8 Lewis, P.J.; Haeusler, G.: Reduction of sympathetic nervous activity as a mechanism of the hypotensive effect of propranolol. Nature *256:* 440 (1975).

9 Management Committee: The Australia therapeutic trial in mild hypertension. Lancet *i:* 1261–1267 (1980).

10 Man In't Veld, A.J.; Schalekamp, M.A.D.H.: How intrinsic sympathomimetic activity modulates the haemodynamic responses to β-adrenoceptor antagonists. A clue to the nature of their antihypertensive mechanism. Br. J. Pharmacol. *13:* suppl., pp. 245–257 (1982).

11 Prichard, B.N.C.: Hypotensive action of pronethalol. Br. med. J. *i:* 1227–1228 (1964).

12 Tung, L.H.; Rand, M.J.; Majewski, H.: Adrenaline-induced hypertension in rats. Clin. Sci. *61:* suppl., pp. 191–193 (1981).

13 Veterans Administration Cooperative Study Group on Hypertension: Effects of treatment on morbidity in hypertension. II. Results in patients with diastolic blood pressure averaging 90 through 114 mm Hg. J. Am. med. Ass. *213:* 1143–1152 (1970).

14 WHO Expert Committee: Arterial hypertension. Technical report series 628 (WHO, Geneva 1978).

15 Zanchetti, A.: Beta-blockers and cardiac involvement in hypertension; in Gross, The cardioprotective action of beta-blockers, pp. 28–37 (Huber, Bern 1977).

16 Zanchetti, A.; Leonetti, G.; Terzoli, L.; Sala, C.: β-Blockers and renin; in Beta-blockers in the 1980s: focus on atenolol. Drugs *25,* suppl. 2, 58S–63S (1983).

Alberto Zanchetti, Center for Clinical Physiology and Hypertension,
University of Milan, I-20122 Milan (Italy)

Angina pectoris and Arrhythmias

Alberto Zanchetti

Milan, Italy

Beta-Blockers in the Treatment of Angina pectoris

Exertional angina, the original indication for which beta-blockers were synthesized and clinically tested [1, 2], is caused by an increased demand for oxygen beyond the limits of a reduced coronary reserve (see part I). Figure 1 shows that noncardioselective – e.g., propranolol and oxprenolol – as well as cardioselective – e.g., practolol, metoprolol, tolamolol – and drugs with – practolol, oxprenolol – or without intrinsic sympathomimetic activity – propranolol, metoprolol, tolamolol – are equally effective in reducing a clinical index of cardiac work, i.e., heart rate-systolic blood pressure product, a reduction clearly evident both at rest and during exercise [19]. Consequently, all beta-blockers effectively increase the treadmill walking time at which angina occurs and reduce the S-T segment depression signalling the onset of exertional angina (fig. 2). Furthermore, the incidence of anginal attacks and the number of glyceryltrinitrate tablets consumed (another index of the incidence of angina) are equally reduced by the different beta-blockers (fig. 3). These data indicate that the antianginal effects of beta-blockers depend on their beta-antagonism and that some degree of intrinsic sympathomimetic activity does not impair their effectiveness. In uncomplicated angina neither cardioselectivity nor intrinsic sympathomimetic activity appears to confer any definite advantage. However, cardioselectivity may be expected to be useful in angina patients with asthma, while intrinsic sympathomimetic activity may be useful in patients with reduced cardiac performance.

The indications for beta-blockers in the treatment of angina at rest are more controversial. If angina at rest is fundamentally due to a sudden re-

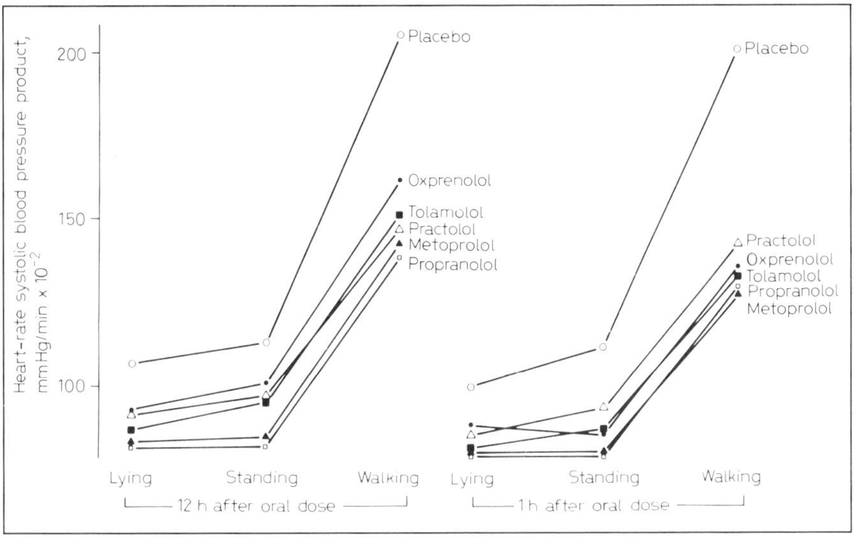

Fig. 1. Comparison of effects of five beta-blockers during sustained treatment in 22 patients with angina pectoris. Data represent mean values. Each of the five drugs reduced the heart rate-systolic blood pressure product with the patient at rest in the supine and standing positions and during exercise compared to the effects of the placebo [from ref. 19, with permission].

duction in myocardial blood flow without any increase in oxygen demand, there is little theoretical basis for a beneficial effect of beta-blockers in this type of angina. Nevertheless, large doses of propranolol have even been reported to be effective in preventing Prinzmetal's variant angina [5], although the most recent therapeutic trend has been toward the use of calcium antagonists in this type of angina [12]. It should not be forgotten, however, that many patients present mixed angina, i.e., anginal episodes during both exertion and at rest. The rationale for using beta-blockers in these patients is readily apparent.

Ischemia-Induced Cardiac Arrhythmias

There are several potential tools for treating and preventing the life-threatening arrhythmias induced by myocardial ischemia – i.e., during the acute stage of myocardial infarction, in unstable angina, or, sometimes, in the ischemic heart in the absence of any other clinical manifestation.

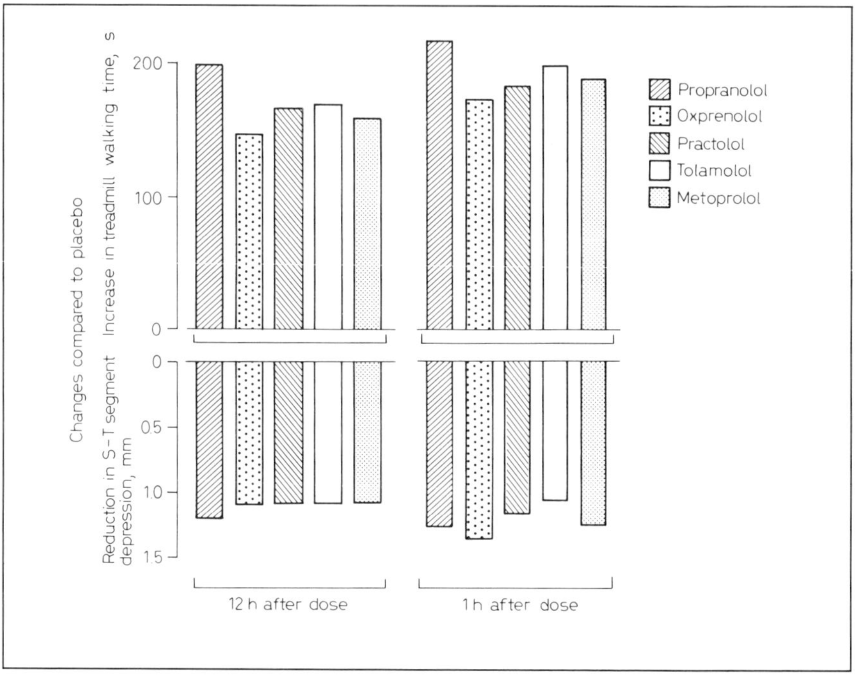

Fig. 2. Comparison of effects of five beta-blockers during sustained treatment in 22 patients with angina pectoris. Data represent mean values. The treadmill walking time to angina was significantly increased, and the S-T segment depression was significantly reduced by each of the five drugs compared to placebo [from ref. 19, with permission].

Adrenergic potentiation of calcium influx through slow channels is a basic factor in reentrant arrhythmias. Consequently, beta-blockers and calcium channel blockers might represent very effective agents in this situation. Beta-blockers and calcium blockers are listed as class II and class IV in the Vaughn-Williams classification of antiarrhythmic drugs.

That beta-adrenergic blockers may be effective in treating or preventing life-threatening arrhythmias in coronary patients is suggested by animal experiments showing a reduction in the number of ventricular dysrhythmias resulting from coronary occlusion [8]. In addition (fig. 4), beta-blockers prevent ventricular fibrillation, when dangerous arrhythmias are precipitated in an animal model by a brief coronary occlusion associated with electrical stimulation of the left stellate ganglion [15].

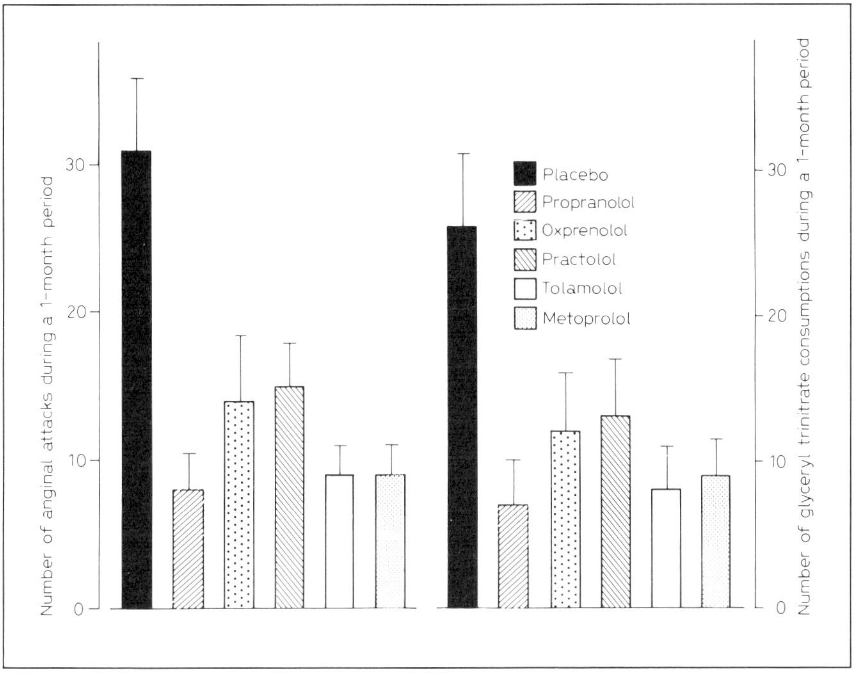

Fig. 3. Comparison of effects of five beta-blockers during sustained treatment in 22 patients with angina pectoris. Data represent mean ± SEM values. The number of anginal attacks and nitroglycerin consumptions were significantly reduced during treatment with each of the five drugs compared to placebo [from ref. 19, with permission].

The effectiveness of beta-blockers in clinical dysrhythmias is less completely documented. In fact, the clinical condition in which prompt administration of beta-adrenergic antagonists may, in principle, be most advantageous – acute myocardial infarction with arrhythmias – generally requires urgent therapeutic measures, precluding studies that satisfy the stringent rules of clinical trials. Most investigators [16, 17], who attempted to treat dysrhythmias during an acute myocardial infarction by administering a beta-blocker intravenously, have found that about 50% of the patients responded favorably. Obviously, the benefit-risk ratio when a beta-blocker is administered under as dangerous a condition as acute myocardial infarction is always difficult to predict and to assess. The outcome in the individual patient will depend largely on the net balance between further depres-

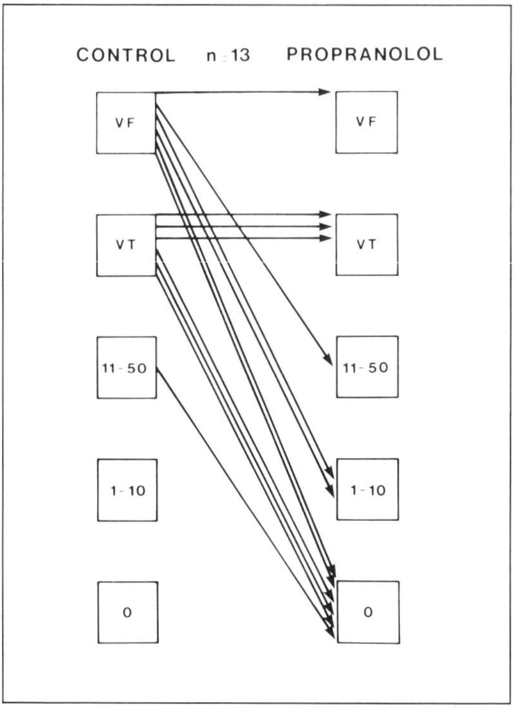

Fig. 4. Effect of propranolol in 13 cats. Each square represents the average result of at least three trials in each cat. The lower squares refer to the number of premature ventricular contractions, the upper squares to ventricular fibrillation (VF) and ventricular tachycardia (VT) [from ref. 15, with permission].

sion of sympathetic-dependent cardiac contractility and a decreased risk of ventricular fibrillation. Encouraging results in the early, but carefully discriminative use of beta-blockers in myocardial infarction have recently been reported in the metoprolol study [6].

The possibility that beta-adrenergic blockers, given early in the course of a myocardial infarction, might help to reduce the size of the infarct has also been explored, mostly in experimental models, with encouraging results [3, 14]. Yet, more must be learned about the effectiveness of beta-blockers in reducing the size of a myocardial infarct in man. This is probably one of the most exciting therapeutic challenges of the 1980s, as the extent of the infarcted area seems to be the most important predictor of subsequent mortality.

On the whole, there appear to be consistent advantages in administering beta-blockers early in the course of myocardial infarction, provided indications are carefully weighed against contraindications. Patients with signs of enhanced sympathetic activity, as shown by *Pantridge* [10] (see also 'Angina pectoris and Cardiac Arrhythmias'), seem to be the most obvious candidates for this therapeutic approach.

The pathophysiologic consideration discussed in 'Angina pectoris and Cardiac Arrhythmias', distinguishing between the mechanisms of early and late arrhythmias in myocardial infarction – i.e., a possibly greater role of reentrant excitation than of enhanced automaticity in early arrhythmias, the reverse being the case for late rhythm disturbances (i.e., those with membrane-stabilizing properties) –, are likely to be somewhat less effective in the first few hours following acute infarction. In fact, there are clinical reports in which lidocaine was found particularly successful in late arrhythmias [11], but not always as effective in earlier arrhythmias [4, 9]. There is evidence, however, that automaticity may also be enhanced by adrenergic hyperactivity [7], suggesting that the use of beta-blockers to moderate this hyperactivity might be of some advantage in late arrhythmias as well.

Finally, minor arrhythmias, such as supraventricular or ventricular ectopic excitations in the presence of a chronic reduction in coronary perfusion, are often responsive to the chronic administration of beta-blockers. These compounds are sometimes more effective and often better tolerated than class I antiarrhythmic agents – i.e., quinidine-like compounds – in the chronic treatment of arrhythmias that, although in themselves of minor hemodynamic significance, may herald more dangerous rhythm disturbances.

Role of Intrinsic Sympathomimetic Activity in the Treatment of Ischemic Heart Disease

Evidence that intrinsic sympathomimetic activity might have some therapeutic advantage is admittedly circumstantial and indirect. Therapeutic advantages in prolonged treatment are necessarily inferred from acute studies [13]. In the management of ischemic heart disease, particularly acute myocardial infarction and life-threatening arrhythmias, actual management is similar to the conditions in experimental studies, making extrapolation easier and more convincing. Intravenous studies in patients with coronary heart disease have shown that beta-blockers with intrinsic sympathomimetic activity, such as oxprenolol and practolol, suppress left ventricular function to a significantly lesser extent than do either propranolol or metoprolol which are devoid of intrinsic sympathomimetic activity [18]. Therefore, beta-blockers with intrinsic sympathomimetic activity appear to maintain cardiac functions more effectively than do drugs without this property when given intravenously to patients with coronary heart disease. As cardiac function tends to be reduced in patients with any manifestation of coronary heart disease, beta-blockers with intrinsic sympathomimetic activity might be a more cautious resource in the treatment of these patients, even when administered orally.

References

1 Alleyns, G.A.O.; Dickinson, C.J.; Dornhorst, A.C.; Fulton, R.M.; Green, K.G.; Hill, T.D.; Hurst, P.; Laurence, D.R.; Pilkington, T.; Prichard, B.N.C.; Robinson, B.; Rosenheim, M.L.: Effect of pronethalol in angina pectoris. Br. med. J. *ii:* 1226–1231 (1963).

2 Black, J.W.; Stephenson, J.S.: Pharmacology of a new adrenergic beta-receptor blocking compound (nethalide). Lancet *ii:* 311–314 (1962).

3 Braunwald, E.; Maroko, P.R.; Libby, P.: Reduction of infarct size following coronary occlusion. Circulation Res. *34–35:* suppl. 3, pp. 192–201 (1974).

4 Darby, S.; Bennett, M.A.; Cruickshank, J.C.; Pentecost, P.L.: Trial of combined intramuscular and intravenous lignocaine in prophylaxis of ventricular tachyarrhythmias. Lancet *i:* 817–819 (1972).

5 Guazzi, M.; Magrini, F.; Fiorentini, C.; Polese, A.: Clinical, electrocardiographic and haemodynamic effects of long term use of propranolol in Prinzmetal's variant angina pectoris. Br. Heart J. *33:* 889–894 (1971).

6 Hjalmarson, A.; Elmfeldt, D.; Herlitz, J.; Holmberg, S.; Malek, I.; Nyberg, G.; Ryden, L.; Swedberg, K.; Vedin, A.; Waagstein, F.; Waldenstrom, A.; Waldenstrom, J.; Wedel, H.; Wilhelmsen, L.; Wilhelmsson, C.: Effect on mortality of metoprolol in acute myocardial infarction. A double-blind randomized trial. Lancet *ii:* 823–827 (1981).

7 Hoffman, B.F.: Role of the sympathetic nervous system in arrhythmias occurring after coronary artery occlusion and myocardial infarction; in Schwartz, Brown, Malliani, Zanchetti, Neural mechanisms in cardiac arrhythmias, pp. 155–166 (Raven Press, New York 1978).

8 Malliani, A.; Schwartz, P.J.; Zanchetti, A.: Neural mechanisms in life-threatening arrhythmias. Am. Heart J. *100:* 705–715 (1980).

9 Pantridge, J.F.: Emergency treatment of cardiac arrhythmias in myocardial infarction; in Scott, Julian, Lidocaine in the treatment of ventricular arrhythmias, pp. 77–81 (Livingstone, Edinburgh 1971).

10 Pantridge, J.F.: Autonomic disturbance at the onset of acute myocardial infarction; in Schwartz, Brown, Malliani, Zanchetti, Neural mechanisms in cardiac arrhythmias, pp. 7–17 (Raven Press, New York 1978).

11 Pantridge, J.F.; Geddes, J.S.: Primary ventricular fibrillation. Eur. J. Cardiol. *1:* 335–339 (1974).
12 Parodi, O.; L'Abbate, A.; Simonetti, I.; Severi, S.; Marzullo, P.; Trivella, M.G.; Maseri, A.: Verapamil in the treatment of vasospastic angina pectoris; in Zanchetti, Krikler, Calcium antagonism in cardiovascular therapy, pp. 176–184 (Excerpta Medica, Amsterdam 1981).
13 Reale, A.; Motolese, M.: Partial agonist activity of beta-adrenergic blocking agents and cardiac performance: a review. Eur. Heart J. *2:* 245–251 (1981).
14 Reimer, K.A.; Rasmussen, M.M.; Jenning, R.B.: On the nature of protection by propranolol against myocardial necrosis after temporary coronary occlusion in dogs. Am. J. Cardiol. *37:* 520–528 (1976).
15 Schwartz, P.J.; Vanoli, E.; Zaza, A.; Zuanetti, G.; Facchini, M.; Pappalettera, M.: The effect of antiarrhythmias induced by interaction between acute myocardial ischemia and sympathetic hyperactivity (to be published).
16 Sloman, G.; Robinson, J.S.; McLean, K.: Propranolol (Inderal) in persistent ventricular fibrillation. Br. med. J. *i:* 895–896 (1965).
17 Taylor, S.H.; Burley, D.M.: Beta-adrenoceptor blocking drugs in post-myocardial infarction dysrhythmias. Proc. R. Soc. Med., suppl. 11, pp. 11–14 (1977).
18 Taylor, S.H.; Silke, B.; Lee, P.S.: Intravenous beta-blockade in coronary heart disease. Is cardioselectivity or intrinsic sympathomimetic activity hemodynamically useful? New Engl. J. Med. *306:* 631–635 (1982).
19 Thadani, U.; Davidson, C.; Singleton, W.; Taylor, S.H.: Comparison of five beta-adrenoreceptor antagonists with different ancillary properties during sustained twice daily therapy in angina pectoris. Am. J. Med. *68:* 243–250 (1980).

Alberto Zanchetti, Center for Clinical Physiology and Hypertension,
University of Milan, I-20122 Milan (Italy)

Psychosomatic Cardiovascular Disorders and Coronary-Prone Behavior

Stevo Julius

Ann Arbor, Mich., USA

Behavioral Treatment

Logically, behavioral treatment should be the appropriate intervention for psychosomatic cardiovascular disorders. Practically, however, it is difficult to demonstrate the usefulness of behavioral treatment. Treatment modes are complex, time consuming, and require repeated return visits to the physician's office. Under such circumstances, it is difficult to include in the evaluation appropriate control groups to differentiate specific effects from those caused by the individual's accommodation to the physician and to office personnel. There is also the question of the placebo effect due to the expectation of improvement. Placebo effects can be significant and long lasting, as has been frequently shown with the placebo effect on blood pressure [11]. Therefore, it is necessary to show that a complex behavioral intervention is more effective than placebo.

Behavioral treatment has most systematically been investigated in hypertension. There are three major categories: biofeedback, relaxation, and meditation. Using biofeedback, *Blanchard* [6], *Goldman* et al. [18], and *Kristt and Engel* [23] reported significant decrements in blood pressure, whereas *Elder and Eustis* [14], *Hager and Surwit* [21], and *Green* et al. [19] failed to find a meaningful effect on the blood pressure. Studies on meditation are less divided. Only *Pollak* et al. [28] found no effect on blood pressure; all other authors report successful results [3, 5, 13, 27, 35]. Even more optimistic are the results with relaxation methods [1, 2, 8, 27]. Approaches, using simultaneous combinations of various methods, have yielded mixed results [4, 12, 16], although a study by *Patel* [27] suggests that an intense combined behavioral treatment strategy may yield sustained blood pressure reductions.

A few generalizations about the overall literature on behavioral treatment of hypertension are possible: (1) Most reports are, in essence, pilot studies, the populations are highly selected, and their numbers are small. (2) Blood pressure effects are modest, generally in the 5- to 10-mm Hg range. (3) Many studies utilized patients already on antihypertensive therapy. The effect of behavioral treatment was then analyzed in terms of a decrease in the number of pills required to control blood pressure. Such results are difficult to evaluate. (4) Rarely has the effect of treatment been evaluated outside of the physician's office or experimental laboratory. It is, therefore, not known whether patients lower their blood pressure on demand in the laboratory or whether the positive effect is extended to daily life. (5) Long-term (years of blood pressure lowering) treatment has not been determined.

Behavioral modification has been suggested for type A coronary-prone individuals. Patients who had already developed a myocardial infarction seem to be most receptive to behavioral modification, and one study provided convincing evidence that the recurrence of symptomatic coronary heart disease events, and even the incidence of deaths, can be reduced by cognitive treatment [29]. Cognitive treatment does not aim to convert a type A to a type B person. This is not a realistic goal for people who developed an entire adult life-style and whose social success, or at least their own perception of social achievements, depended on that life-style. Stress management techniques do not appear to be effective for the treatment of type A behavior [22]. *Chesney and Rosenman* [10] and *Rosenman and Friedman* [31] underscore the trichotomy of type A behavior; the expression of the syndrome depends on emotional and behavioral components, environmental stressors, and the subject's interpretation and responses to these stressors. Their cognitive therapy [10, 31] takes into consideration all of these elements and also uses adjunct methods of muscular relaxation and general arousal reduction. Whether behavioral treatment can prevent the development of myocardial infarction in a primary fashion remains to be seen. Modifying a type A individuals' coping styles [32] resulted in an improved feeling of well-being and improved productivity [33]. Even if proven effective, cognitive treatment of type A behavior is not applicable on a large scale and, therefore, is not likely to have a major impact on type A related coronary morbidity.

Pharmacologic Treatment

Underlying all psychosomatic cardiovascular manifestations in hypertension, in type A behavior, and in ventricular arrhythmias are periods of intensive sympathetic cardiac activation. This excess sympathetic drive is associated with a tachycardiac response to environmental stressors. Excessive beta-adrenergic drive to the heart is viewed as an important factor in the pathophysiology of coronary heart disease in type A individuals [30] and in the pathophysiology of increased cardiac vulnerability to arrhythmias [25]. The role of these heart rate oscillations in the pathophysiology of hypertension is not elucidated, but it is of interest to note that transient tachycardia, even in normotensive individuals, is a predictor of future hypertension and of hypertensive cardiovascular morbidity [24]. *Carruthers* [9] proposed a unifying hypothesis of how excess catecholamines during emotional stress leads both to excessive swings in blood pressure and to the formation of atheroma in coronary vasculature. Higher catecholamine excretion tends to mobilize free fatty acids which may be transformed in the liver to triglycerides and cholesterol. Raised free fatty acids are also arrhythmogenic. This excess noradrenergic drive leads to a formation of the substrate for both the development of coronary atheroma and for sudden death. *Michael* [26] and *Taggart and Carruthers* [36] have demonstrated that oxprenolol effectively prevents blood pressure, lipid, and electrocardiographic signs of emotion in stressful situations. Prevention (using oxprenolol) of lypolysis under mental stress has been elegantly demonstrated by *Taylor* [37, 38] who showed that psychosomatic effects on the heart are predominantly beta-adrenergic and, therefore, should be readily abolished by beta-adrenergic blockade. The specificity of beta-blocking agents in psychosomatic cardiac disorders has been shown by *Braathen* et al. [7] who found that alprenolol is more effective than placebo in preventing palpitations and tremor in patients with neurocirculatory asthenia. Such nonspecific symptoms as cardiac pain and dyspnea have not been significantly more reduced with alprenolol than with placebo.

The specificity of beta-blocking agents in reducing tachycardia and palpitations may prove to be therapeutically important. Emotion-inducing behaviors are invariably associated with cardiovascular response, but the opposite is also true: that cardiovascular reactions have an influence on emotions. This point of ‘reinforcement’ of emotional responses by their cardiovascular manifestations has been extensively documented in the psychosomatic literature. An example is the study by *Valin* [39] in which individuals were more apt to report they became excited by a nude picture, if a display on the screen suggested that they also had tachycardia. This induction of emotional responses is clearly beta-adrenergic. *Frohlich* et al. [17] elicited anxiety attacks with isoproterenol infusion in patients with a hyper-beta-adrenergic syndrome, but such attacks could not be elicited if tachycardia was caused by atropine. *Guazzi* et al. [20] have shown the clinical usefulness of beta-adrenergic blockade in such patients.

The specific properties of beta-blocking agents – (1) they abolish the metabolic effects of the hypersympathetic state; (2) they abolish electrocardiographic changes in response to emotion, and (3) they abolish secondary emotional responses to tachycardia and palpitations – make them particularly suitable for the treatment of psychosomatic cardiovascular disorders. Tranquilizers are much less specific and, therefore, less useful in the treatment of psychosomatic cardiovascular manifestations.

There is another interesting aspect of the action of beta-blocking agents that may be useful in the treatment of type A behavior: there are clear behavioral changes in patients on beta-adrenergic blockade. Every observant clinician has found that patients on beta-blockade are less high-strung, less bothered by deadlines, and are frequently better organized under pressure. This specific 'anti-type A' effect should be differentiated from the well-documented anxiolytic effect of beta-blocking agents [15]. A recent preliminary report suggests that the clinical impression about the beneficial effects of beta-blockade on type A behavior may be correct. *Schmieder* et al. [34] found that type A individuals moved toward type B behavior on beta-blockade, whereas patients on diuretics moved in the opposite direction. This effect of beta-blocking agents opens a whole new field of pharmacologic intervention into type A behavior, using drugs that prevent cardiovascular complications while possibly also altering basic behavior.

One of the undesired side effects of beta-blockade is decreased cardiac performance with the attendant symptom of tiredness and decreased exercise performance. Beta-blocking agents with intrinsic sympathomimetic activity have fewer of these side effects as the heart rate at rest is not reduced and exercise performance at lower levels of load is not impaired. If one also considers the known cardioprotective effect of oxprenolol against the recurrence of myocardial infarction, which will be discussed in 'The Postmyocardial Infarction Patient', oxprenolol appears to offer a very acceptable and proven mode of intervention in coronary-prone patients as well as in those who suffer from functional cardiovascular disorders.

References

1 Bali, L.R.: Long-term effect of relaxation on blood pressure and anxiety levels of essential hypertensive males: a controlled study. Psychosom. Med. *41:* 637–646 (1979).

2 Beimann, I.; Graham, L.E.; Ciminero, A.R.: Self-control progressive relaxation training as an alternative nonpharmacological treatment of essential hypertension: therapeutic effects in the natural environment. Behav. Res. Therapy *16:* 371–375 (1978).

3 Benson, H.; Rosner, B.A.; Marzetta, B.R.; Klemchuck, H.M.: Decreased blood pressure in pharmacologically treated hypertensive patients who regularly elicited the relaxation response. Lancet *i:* 289–291 (1974).

4 Bertilson, H.S.: Treatment program for borderline hypertension among college students: relaxation, finger temperature, biofeedback, and generalization. Psychol. Rep. *44:* 107–114 (1979).

5 Blackwell, B.: Transcendental meditation in hypertension: individual response patterns. Lancet *i:* 223–226 (1976).

6 Blanchard, E.B.: A simple feedback system for the treatment of elevated blood pressure. Behav. Ther. *6:* 241–245 (1975).

7 Braathen, L.R.; Gisholt, K.; Helkbo, R.; Schroder, P.; Svendsen, E.R.; Albrektsen, T.: Effect of alprenolol in patients with neurocirculatory asthenia: a controlled double-blind study in general practice. Pharmatherapeutica *1:* 381–388 (1977).

8 Brauer, A.P.; Horlick, L.; Nelson, E.; Farquhar, J.W.; Agras, W.S.: Relaxation therapy for essential hypertension: a Veterans Administration outpatient study. J. behav. Med. *2:* 21–29 (1979).

9 Carruthers, M.: Aggression and atheroma. Lancet *ii:* 1170–1171 (1969).

10 Chesney, M.A.; Rosenman, R.H.: Strategies for modifying type A behavior. Consultant *1980:* 216–222.

11 Cottier, C.; Julius, S.; Gajendragadkar, S.V.; Schork, M.A.: Usefulness of home BP determination in treating borderline hypertension. J. Am. med. Ass. *248:* 555–558 (1982).

12 Datey, K.K.: Role of biofeedback training in hypertension and stress. J. postgrad. Med. *26:* 68–73 (1980).

13 Datey, K.K.; Desmukh, S.N.; Dalvi, C.P.; Vinekar, S.L.: 'Shavasen': a yogic exercise in the management of hypertension. Angiology *20:* 325–333 (1969).

14 Elder, S.T.; Eustis, N.K.: Instrumental blood pressure conditioning in outpatient hypertensives. Behav. Res. Therapy *13:* 185–188 (1975).

15 Elsdon-Dew, R.W.: Clinical trials of oxprenolol in anxiety. Scot. med. J. *20:* 286–287 (1975).

16 Frankel, B.L.; Patel, D.J.; Horwitz, D.; Friedewald, D.T.; Gaardner, K.R.: Treatment of hypertension with biofeedback and relaxation techniques. Psychosom. Med. *40:* 276–293 (1979).

17 Frohlich, E.D.; Tarazi, R.C.; Dustan, H.P.: Hyperdynamic beta-adrenergic circulatory state: increased beta-receptor responsiveness. Archs intern. Med. *123:* 1–7 (1969).

18 Goldman, H.; Kleinmann, K.; Snow, M.; Bidus, D.; Korol, B.: Relationship between essential hypertension and cognitive functioning: effect of biofeedback. Psychophysiology *12:* 569–573 (1975).

19 Green, E.E.; Green, A.M.; Norris, P.A.: Self-regulation training for control of hypertension. Prim. Cardiol. *6:* 126–137 (1980).
20 Guazzi, M.; Polese, A.; Magrini, F.; Fiorentini, C.; Olivari, M.T.: Long-term treatment of the hyperkinetic heart syndrome with propranolol. Am. J. med. Sci. *270:* 465–474 (1975).
21 Hager, J.L.; Surwit, R.S.: Hypertension self-control with a portable feedback unit or meditation-relaxation. Biofeedback Self-Regul. *3:* 269–276 (1978).
22 Jenni, M.A.; Wollersheim, J.P.: Cognitive therapy, stress management training and the type A behavior pattern. Cognitive Ther. Res. *3:* 61–73 (1979).
23 Kristt, D.A.; Engel, B.T.: Learned control of blood pressure in patients with high blood pressure. Circulation *51:* 370–378 (1975).
24 Levy, R.L.; White, P.D.; Stroud, W.D.; Hillman, C.C.: Transient tachycardia: prognostic significance alone and in association with transient hypertension. J. Am. med. Ass. *129:* 585–588 (1945).
25 Lown, B.: Mental stress, arrhythmias and sudden death. Am. J. Med. *72:* 177–180 (1982).
26 Michael, J.: A placebo-controlled double-blind trial of oxprenolol versus diazepam in the treatment of anxiety and stress; in Kielholz, Siegenthaler, Taggart, Zanchetti, Psychosomatic cardiovascular disorders – when and how to treat?, pp. 191–196 (Huber, Bern 1981).
27 Patel, C.H.: Twelve-month follow-up of yoga and biofeedback in the management of hypertension. Lancet *i:* 62–65 (1975).
28 Pollak, A.D.; Weber, M.A.; Case, D.B.; Laragh, J.H.: Limitations of transcendental meditation in the treatment of essential hypertension. Lancet *i:* 71–73 (1977).
29 Rahe, R.H.; Ward, H.W.; Hayes, V.: Brief group therapy in myocardial infarction rehabilitation: three to four-year follow-up of a controlled trial. Psychosom. Med. *41:* 229–242 (1979).
30 Rosenman, R.H.; Chesney, M.A.: Psychological profiles and coronary heart disease; in Kielholz, Siegenthaler, Taggart, Zanchetti, Psychosomatic cardiovascular disorders – when and how to treat?, pp. 37–50 (Huber, Bern 1981).
31 Rosenman, R.H.; Friedman, M.: Modifying type A behavior pattern. J. psychosom. Res. *21:* 323–331 (1977).
32 Roskies, E.; Kearney, H.; Spevack, M.; Surkis, A.; Cohen, C.; Gilman, S.: Generalizability and durability of treatment effects in an intervention program for coronary-prone (type A) managers. J. behav. Med. *2:* 195–207 (1979).
33 Roskies, E.; Lazarus, R.S.: Coping therapy and the teaching of coping skills; in Davidson, Behavioral medicine: changing health life styles (Brunner/Mazel, New York 1980).
34 Schmieder, R.; Friedrich, G.; Neus, H.; Ruddel, H.; Eiff, A.W. von: The influence of beta-blocker on cardiovascular reactivity and type A behavior pattern in hypertensives. Am. Psychosom. Soc. Annu. Meet., Denver 1982.
35 Stone, R.A.; DeLeo, J.: Psychotherapeutic control of hypertension. New Engl. J. Med. *294:* 80–84 (1976).
36 Taggart, P.; Carruthers, M.: Suppression by oxprenolol of adrenergic response to stress. Lancet *ii:* 256–258 (1972).

37 Taylor, S.H.: Stress, cardiovascular disease, and beta-adrenoceptor antagonists; in Kielholz, Beta-blockers and the central nervous system. Int. Symp., St. Moritz 1976, p. 90 (Huber, Bern 1977).
38 Taylor, S.H.: Stress, hypertension, and ischaemic heart disease; in Kielholz, Siegenthaler, Taggart, Zanchetti, Psychosomatic cardiovascular disorders – when and how to treat?, pp. 120–137 (Huber, Bern 1981).
39 Valin, S.: The perception and labeling of bodily changes as determinants of emotional behavior; in Black, Physiologic correlates of emotion, p. 299 (Academic Press, New York 1970).

Stevo Julius, Division of Hypertension, Department of Internal Medicine, University of Michigan School of Medicine, Ann Arbor, MI 48109 (USA)

The Postmyocardial Infarction Patient

Alberto Zanchetti
Milan, Italy

Beta-Blockers in Secondary Prevention of Myocardial Infarction

Myocardial infarction is traditionally regarded as a thromboembolic disease, although other factors are known to be involved. Therefore, attempts have been made in several studies to interfere with thromboembolic and related processes by administering (1) plasma lipid lowering substances; (2) anticoagulant drugs, and (3), more recently, antiplatelet agents.

Another secondary prophylactic approach has been followed by other investigators. As discussed in 'Angina pectoris and Cardiac Arrhythmias', life-threatening arrhythmias often occur in the acutely ischemic myocardium. The role played by sympathetic cardiac innervation in facilitating these arrhythmias has led to the use of beta-blockers in their treatment in coronary patients. These same considerations explain why various beta-blockers have been used in approximately 25 trials from 1965 to the present in order to prevent sudden death and reinfarction in patients who had suffered a previous myocardial infarction [9]. The various trials and the beta-blocking agents used are listed in table I.

For many years, the results of these trials have been disappointing and contradictory. Until 1977, the Multicentre International Study on practolol [6] was the primary source of evidence for the role of beta-blockers in secondary prevention. This trial showed a statistically significant 38% reduction in total mortality and also a significant reduction in sudden death. Benefits were concentrated almost exclusively in patients who had suffered an anterior myocardial infarction. However, most studies up to 1981, although they showed a general trend toward benefits from beta-blockers,

Table I. Beta-blockers used in secondary prevention trials of myocardial infarction

Beta-blocker	Number of trials	References [cited in ref. 9]
Propranolol	10	*Snow,* 1965 *Balcon* et al., 1966 *Clausen* et al., 1966 Multicentre trial, 1966 *Barber* et al., 1967 *Norris* et al., 1968 *Barber* et al., 1980 *Wilcox, Roland* et al., 1980 *Hansteen* et al., 1982 Beta-Blocker Heart Attack Study Group, 1982
Alprenolol	4	*Reynolds and Whitlock,* 1972 *Wilhelmsson* et al., 1974 *Ahlmark and Saetre,* 1976 *Andersen* et al., 1979
Practolol	2	Multicentre International Study, 1975, 1977 *Barber* et al., 1975
Oxprenolol	3	*Wilcox, Rowley* et al., 1980 Coronary Prevention Research Group, 1981 *Taylor* et al., 1982
Atenolol	1	*Wilcox, Roland* et al., 1980
Timolol	1	Norwegian Multicentre Study Group, 1981
Metoprolol	3	*Rehnquist* et al., 1980 *Hjalmarson* et al., 1981 *McIlmoyle* et al., 1981
Sotalol	1	*Julian* et al., 1982

provided, on the whole, contradictory and inconclusive results. In contrast, during 1981 and 1982, data from several trials indicated that treatment with beta-blockers may indeed provide benefits in the secondary prevention of myocardial infarction and cardiac death.

The Norwegian Multicentre Study Group [7], in 1,884 patients, reported a timolol-induced 39% reduction in mortality, a 44% reduction in sudden death, and a 28% reduction in reinfarction during an average observation period of 33 months. All of these reductions were statistically significant. In a subsequent study by *Hjalmarson* et al. [3], either a placebo or metoprolol was given intravenously to 1,395 patients shortly after they arrived in the hospital. Patients were then maintained on oral doses of these medications for 90 days. At the end of the 3-month study period, the mortality was 36% lower in the metoprolol-treated group, a statistically significant difference.

Favorable results have also been reported in two recent trials in which propranolol has been used. In the Norwegian study by *Hansteen* et al. [2] 560 patients, all of whom had severe arrhythmias or left ventricular failure at the time of infarction and were considered at high risk, were randomly allocated to either propranolol or placebo. After 1 year of medication, the propranolol-treated group had a 31% reduction in total mortality, a 51% reduction in sudden death, and a 25% reduction in reinfarction. However, only the decrease in sudden death was statistically significant. In the largest published trial, the Beta-Blocker Heart Attack Trial Research Group [1], 3,837 patients were randomly allocated to receive either propranolol or placebo. The propranolol-treated group had statistically significant reductions in total mortality (26%) and in sudden cardiac death (28%). As in all recent trials, benefits were seen in both anterior and inferior infarctions.

The sotalol trial [4] has recently given less satisfactory results, as the beta-blocker reduced total mortality by only 18%, a statistically nonsignificant reduction. Also in this trial, a statistically significant 41% reduction in the reinfarction rate was observed in patients treated with sotalol. Finally, oxprenolol in a recently completed study [8] also provided benefits, but these were limited to patients whose treatment was started within 4 months from the time of myocardial infarction. Treatment started more than 1 year from the time of myocardial infarction appeared to produce more disadvantages than advantages (see also 'Clinical Results').

Lewis [5] recently surveyed the 17 most important secondary prevention studies using beta-blockers, both studies that had showed significant differences and those that individually seemed more inconclusive. Pooled analyses of all 17 trials indicate a statistically significant reduction in mortality in the beta-blocker treated group, averaging 21% with 95% confidence limits ranging from 13 to 28%. Thus, both the upper and lower confidence limits of the beta-blocker effect were on the benefit side (fig. 1). There was no evidence of heterogeneity of the treatment effect – i.e., results of individual trials were consistent. The analysis trials by *Lewis* [5] have also been classified as early or late interventions, based on a 48-hour cutoff between the onset of symptoms and the beginning of treatment. The pooled

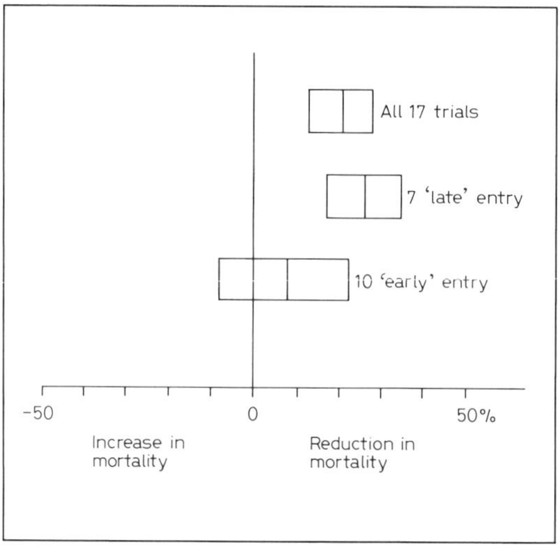

Fig. 1. Effects of beta-blockers on postinfarction mortality. Pooled results for 17 trials with 95% confidence limits [from ref. 5, with permission].

results of the seven late-entry trials show a highly significant positive effect, the average reduction in mortality being 26% with 95% confidence limits of 17–35% (fig. 1). On the other hand, analysis of the 10 early-entry trials shows a small positive effect, with an average reduction in mortality of 8%, with 95% confidence intervals ranging from −8 to 22% (fig. 1). This small reduction had no statistical or clinical significance.

It can, therefore, be concluded that beta-blockers play a useful role in the secondary prevention of myocardial infarction. The fact that benefits have been observed with a variety of beta-adrenergic blockers, with or without membrane-stabilizing or intrinsic sympathomimetic activity or beta-1-selectivity, suggests that protection may indeed be due to blockade of sympathetic influences on the heart. An important problem remains, however; that is, the best time for starting beta-blocker administration, whether as early as possible after the onset of pain or a few days thereafter, when the patient has recovered from the acute phase. Pathophysiologic considerations suggest early intervention, because adrenergic activity plays a particularly noxious role in the early hours, facilitating life-threatening arrhythmias and extending the infarction area. Early intervention is not without complications, however – excessive bradycardia, atrioventricular block, pump failure, and so on –, and the balance of benefits and risks can only be established for the individual patient.

The success of the metoprolol study [3] indicates that early intervention by an expert cardiologist can favorably overcome these difficulties. The positive results of the metoprolol study must be looked at critically, however, in view of the less favorable indications resulting from the pooled analysis of several early-entry as compared with several late-entry trials [5]. Clearly, there is an urgent need for more information about early interventions.

Role of Intrinsic Sympathomimetic Activity in Secondary Prevention of Myocardial Infarction

Favorable prophylactic results have been obtained with several beta-blockers with different additional properties. Intrinsic sympathomimetic activity is certainly unnecessary for these favorable effects which have been induced by propranolol, timolol, and metoprolol, all drugs devoid of intrinsic sympathomimetic activity. This activity, however, does not prevent the favorable effects, inasmuch as positive results have also been observed with oxprenolol, practolol, and alprenolol. Furthermore, there is no proof that intrinsic sympathomimetic activity is of further prophylactic value, although it has been argued that beta-blockers with this activity might be a more cautious form of treatment for coronary heart disease, especially in patients with acute myocardial infarction. Early intravenous injection of beta-blockers in these patients may limit the extent of infarction and provides a protective effect during the most dangerous early hours. Thus, early intervention, using compounds with intrinsic sympathomimetic activity, should be tested further.

References

1 Beta-Blocker Heart Attack Trial Research Group: a randomized trial of propranolol in patients with acute myocardial infarction. I. Mortality results. J. Am. med. Ass. *247:* 1707–1714 (1982).

2 Hansteen, V.; Moinichen, E.; Lorentsen, E.; Andersen, A.; Strom, O.; Soiland, K.; Dyrbekk, D.; Refsum, A.M.; Tromsdal, A.; Knodsen, K.; Eika, C.; Bakken, J.; Smith, P.; Hoff, P.I.: One year's treatment with propranolol after myocardial infarction: preliminary report of Norwegian Multicentre Trial. Br. med. J. *284:* 155–160 (1982).

3 Hjalmarson, A.; Elmfeldt, D.; Herlitz, J.; Holmberg, S.; Malek, I.; Nyberg, G.; Ryden, L.; Swedberg, K.; Vedin, A.; Waagstein, F.; Waldestrom, A.; Wilhelmsen, L.; Wilhelmsson, C.: Effect of mortality of metoprolol in acute myocardial infarction. Lancet *ii:* 823–827 (1981).
4 Julian, D.G.; Prescott, R.J.; Jackson, F.S.; Szekely, P., et al.: A controlled trial of sotalol for one year after myocardial infarction. Lancet *i:* 1142–1147 (1982).
5 Lewis, J.A.: β-Blockade after myocardial infarction. A statistical view. Br. J. clin. Pharmacol. *14:* suppl., pp. 15–21 (1982).
6 Multicentre International Study: supplementary report. Reduction in mortality after myocardial infarction with long-term beta-adrenoreceptor blockade. Br. med. J. *ii:* 419–421 (1977).
7 Norwegian Multicentre Study Group: Timolol-induced reduction in mortality and reinfarction in patients surviving acute myocardial infarction. New Engl. J. Med. *304:* 801–807 (1981).
8 Taylor, S.H.; Silke, B.; Ebbutt, A.; Sutton, G.C.; Prout, B.J.; Burley, D.M.: A long-term prevention study with oxprenolol in coronary heart disease. New Engl. J. Med. *307:* 1294–1301 (1982).
9 Zanchetti, A.: Treatment with beta-adrenoreceptor blockers in secondary prevention of myocardial infarction; in Secondary prevention of ischemic cardiac events (Huber, Bern 1983).

Alberto Zanchetti, Center for Clinical Physiology and Hypertension,
University of Milan, I-20122 Milan (Italy)

III. Oxprenolol (®Trasicor) – Scientific Profile

Pharmacology

Jacob V. Aranda

Montreal, Que., Canada

Introduction

Alpha- and Beta-Adrenergic Receptor Concept

Pharmacologists have developed special concepts to explain the relationship between chemical structure and the resulting pharmacologic action of a drug.

With certain exceptions, most drugs produce their effects by combining with enzymes, cell membranes, or other specialized components of cells. Such drug-cell interaction alters the function of the cell component, initiating the series of biochemical and physiologic changes by which the drug is identified and characterized. The cell component directly involved in the action of the drug is usually termed its receptive substance or, simply, its receptor. The formation of the drug-receptor complex, the initial action of the drug, and the early events in the action-effects sequence are sometimes referred to collectively as the receptor process.

The concept of receptors was developed at the beginning of this century by *Dale, Langley,* and *Ehrlich,* but it was more than 40 years later that this concept was first applied to the sympathetic nervous system.

In 1948, Dr. *Raymond P. Ahlquist* [1], Professor of Pharmacology at the Medical College of Georgia, advanced a theory based on his investigations into the effects exerted on the heart, smooth muscle, and peripheral blood vessels by the two naturally occurring transmitter substances epinephrine and norepinephrine as well as by three synthetic catecholamines. He had found that, depending on the effector organ concerned, the various catecholamines differed in the relative potency of their activity. Epinephrine and norepinephrine, for example, produced the strongest vasoconstrictive effect on peripheral blood vessels, whereas the synthetic catecholamine isoproterenol proved to be the weakest in this respect. When the five sub-

Table I. Responses of effector organs to adrenergic impulses [from ref. 10]

Effector organs	Adrenergic impulses	
	receptor type	responses[a]
Heart		
S-A node	β_1	increase in heart rate ++
Atria	β_1	increase in contractility and conduction velocity ++
A-V node	β_1	increase in automaticity and conduction velocity ++
His-Purkinje system	β_1	increase in automaticity and conduction velocity +++
Ventricles	β_1	increase in contractility, conduction velocity, automaticity, and rate of idioventricular pacemakers +++
Arterioles		
Coronary	α, β_2	constriction +; dilation ++[b]
Skin and mucosa	α	constriction +++
Skeletal muscle	α, β_2	constriction ++; dilation ++[b, c]
Cerebral	α	constriction (slight)
Pulmonary	α, β_2	constriction +; dilation[b]
Abdominal viscera, renal	α, β_2	constriction +++; dilation +[c]
Salivary glands	α	constriction +++
Veins (systemic)	α, β_2	constriction ++; dilation ++
Lung		
Bronchial muscle	β_2	relaxation +
Kidney	β_2	renin secretion ++
Pancreas		
Acini	α	decreased secretion +
Islets (β-cells)	α	decreased secretion +++
	β_2	increased secretion +
Fat cells	α, β_1	lipolysis +++[d]

[a] Responses are designated + to +++ to provide an approximate indication of the importance of adrenergic nerve activity in the control of the various organs and functions listed.
[b] Dilation predominates in situ due to metabolic autoregulatory phenomena.
[c] Over the usual concentration range of physiologically released, circulating epinephrine, *beta*-receptor response (vasodilation) predominates in blood vessels of skeletal muscle and liver; *alpha*-receptor response (vasoconstriction) in blood vessels of other abdominal viscera. The renal and mesenteric vessels also contain specific dopaminergic receptors, activation of which causes dilation, but their physiologic significance has not been established.
[d] The type of receptor mediating certain metabolic responses varies significantly among species.

stances were classified by reference to the extent to which they increased the heart rate, isoproterenol emerged as the most effective and norepinephrine as the least effective. In the light of these observations, *Ahlquist* [1] postulated that the differing degrees of activity displayed by catecholamines in one effector organ as compared with another must be due to the existence of two different types of receptor which he arbitrarily named *alpha* and *beta.*

This concept was later amplified by subdividing the beta receptors into beta-1- and beta-2-receptors (table I). The significance of *Ahlquist's* hypothesis was confirmed when a substance was discovered which specifically blocked beta-adrenergic reactions in the effector organs, namely, dichloroisoproterenol. This substance proved too toxic for therapeutic use, but subsequently other substances were found capable of exerting a clinically useful beta-adrenergic inhibiting effect. The term 'beta-blocker', however, should, strictly speaking, be applied only to those substances which specifically antagonize endogenous or exogenous beta-stimulation. Since their discovery, the beta-blockers have gained widespread acceptance for the treatment of a wide range of cardiovascular disorders, such as hypertension, angina pectoris, and disturbances of cardiac rhythm.

Although all beta-blockers have an inhibitory effect on beta-adrenergic receptors, they differ in the presence or absence of additional pharmacologic properties such as membrane-stabilizing activity, intrinsic sympathomimetic activity, and cardioselectivity.

The following pages will present a summarized overview of the distinctive chemistry and pharmacokinetic and pharmacodynamic properties of the beta-adrenoceptor blocker oxprenolol, its range of indications, and dosage recommendations.

Chemistry

Oxprenolol (®Trasicor) is the hydrochloride of the racemic form of 1-(*o*-allyloxyphenoxy)-3-(isopropylamino)-2-propanol, with a molecular weight of 301.81. Figure 1 represents the structural formula. The salt is readily water soluble (70 g/100 ml water). The optical antipodes of oxprenolol display the properties typical of this class of drugs, i.e., the (–)-isomer is about twice as potent as an antagonist of cardiac beta-adrenoceptors as the racemate, whereas the (+)-isomer is considerably less active [3, 15]. The pH value of a 1% aqueous solution is 6.0. Oxprenolol is also soluble in methanol, ethanol, and chloroform. The melting point is 107 °C.

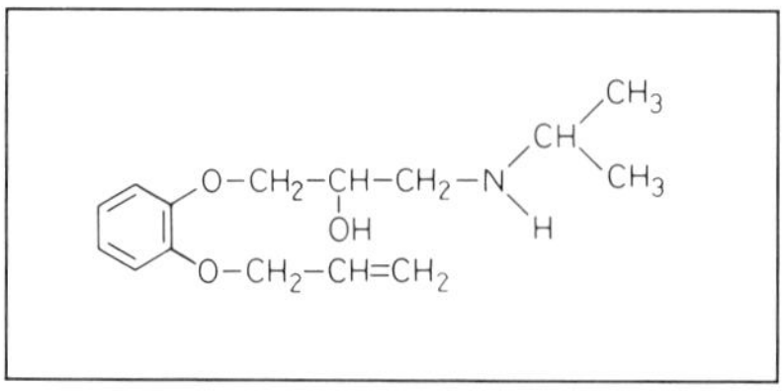

Fig. 1. Structure. Molecular formula: $C_{15}H_{23}NO_3HCl$.

Oxprenolol has a pKa value of 9.5. It is less lipophilic than propranolol. Partition coefficients between octanol and buffer are 0.43 at pH 7 and 4.11 at pH 8, whereas the partition coefficients of propranolol are 5.39 and 52.5 at the same pH values [3, 11]. Partition coefficients between chloroform and water are 8.09 for oxprenolol and 15.67 for propranolol [3, 20].

Pharmacokinetics

Absorption, Distribution, Bioavailability, and Excretion

Animal and human studies have shown that oxprenolol is rapidly and almost completely absorbed [18, 19]. After oral administration of radioactively labelled oxprenolol, 70–100% of the administered dose was eliminated in the urine of healthy volunteers within 48 h [18, 19]. When oxprenolol is administered orally, peak plasma concentrations of the unchanged active substance are generally attained within 30 min to 1 h. Oxprenolol is absorbed to the same extent from sustained-release formulations [17, 21]. Here, however, peak plasma concentrations are not achieved for several hours (fig. 2) and are lower than following the same dose given in a conventional formulation. Between 4 and 12 h after administration of the sustained-release formulation the plasma concentrations are appreciably higher than those attained by conventional formulations (fig. 2). Chronic administration has no effect on the disposition kinetics of oxprenolol. No accumulation of oxprenolol with doses up to 80 mg three times daily has been observed [5].

In rat studies using labelled oxprenolol, the highest total activities were found in the liver, kidney, lung, and heart [13]. Oxprenolol is approximately 80% protein bound in human plasma [17], whereas propranolol is approximately 93% protein bound [8].

Like propranolol, oxprenolol is extensively metabolized. With both beta-blockers, biotransformation proceeds along the same principal path-

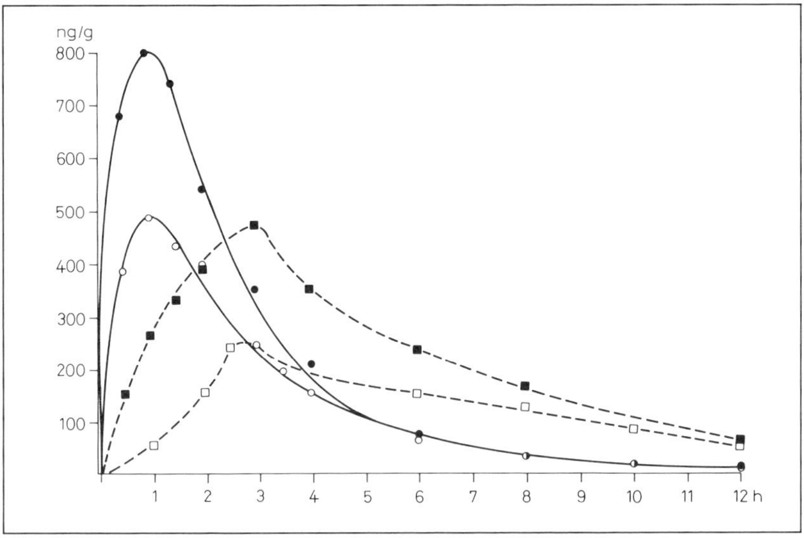

Fig. 2. Average oxprenolol concentration curves in plasma of 6 healthy volunteers after single oral doses of 80 mg Trasicor (○), 80 mg Trasicor slow release (□), 160 mg Trasicor (●), and 160 mg Trasicor slow release (■) [17].

ways [9, 13] involving *o*- and N-dealkylation, oxidation of the propanolamine side chain, aromatic hydroxylation, and glucuronidation.

Dawes et al. [7] studied the influence of food on plasma levels of conventional and slow-release oxprenolol in healthy volunteers. They observed no significant trends in plasma drug profiles due to food with either formulation. Elimination half-lives were longer after food with conventional tablets, presumably owing to continued absorption. These investigators state that slow-release oxprenolol, under the conditions of their study, was shown to be a reliable and convenient dosage form providing similar plasma-drug profiles in fasted and nonfasted subjects [7].

Studies in man have revealed that the pharmacokinetics of oxprenolol differ from the pharmacokinetics of other beta-adrenergic antagonists. A first-pass effect has been observed with oxprenolol. The systemic bioavailability of oxprenolol was reported by *Mason and Winer* [14] to be 19–74%, and by *Kendall* et al. [12] to be 25–30%; in both instances the determinations were made in 6 healthy volunteers. The systemic bioavailability, however, is not dose dependent, but varies in different individuals and is fairly reproducible within an individual over the dosage range of 20–160 mg [14].

Although oxprenolol has a relatively short half-life, as do the other highly metabolized drugs in this class, its half-life varies neither with the dose nor with the route of administration, indicating that at plasma concentrations in the therapeutic range, distribution and elimination of oxprenolol occur by linear rate processes [14].

Hemodynamic, Cardiac, and Peripheral Circulatory Effects

Oxprenolol is a nonselective beta-adrenoceptor antagonist. It affects both beta-1-organs, e.g., the heart, and beta-2-organs, e.g., the blood vessels [2, 4, 16]. In addition to its beta-antagonist effects, oxprenolol also exerts a moderate partial agonist action on the beta-adrenoceptors, referred to as 'intrinsic sympathomimetic activity'.

These properties as well as other hemodynamic, cardiac, and peripheral circulatory effects are fully described in 'Clinical Results'. For further details relevant to the pharmacodynamics of oxprenolol, see *Brechbühler* et al. [3].

Toxicity

Animal Studies

As is evident from the data summarized below, one of the distinctive features of oxprenolol is its moderate to low degree of toxicity [6].

Acute Toxicity

The LD_{50} for oxprenolol is 30 ± 3 mg/kg i.v. and 245 ± 40 mg/kg s.c. in mice. In rats, the LD_{50} values for oxprenolol are 33 ± 3 mg/kg i.v., 940 ± 58 mg/kg s.c., and 730 ± 48 mg/kg orally.

Chronic Toxicity

No toxic effects were observed in rats treated with oxprenolol for 12 months in daily oral doses of 30 mg/kg. At 100 mg/kg per day, the growth rate of male rats declined; liver weights were slightly increased, but no histologic changes were noted. Doses of 300 mg/kg oxprenolol orally caused death.

Oral doses of 10 and 30 mg/kg daily administered to dogs for 6 months elicited no demonstrable toxic effects. At doses of 200 and 300 mg/kg per day, the growth rate of female dogs decreased somewhat; serum alkaline phosphatase levels were elevated, and liver weights were significantly increased although no histologic changes were evident.

Oral doses of 15 and 50 mg/kg for 12 months also caused no toxic manifestations in dogs. With 150 mg/kg per day, an increased incidence of vomiting and salivation was noted with signs of central nervous system stimulation. These effects disappeared, when the daily dosage was given in two divided doses. Results of biochemical, hematologic, macroscopic, and microscopic studies disclosed no evidence of toxic changes.

Effects on Reproduction

Oxprenolol in oral doses up to 150 mg/kg did not affect the fertility of male rats. The reproductive capacity of female rats was normal as was parturition and the growth and development of the newborn. No untoward effects occurred in pregnant or lactating dams treated with oxprenolol in oral doses of 150 mg/kg. The only effect of these high doses on the fetus was slightly less body weight gain during late pregnancy. The survival of sucklings was not affected.

Studies of Teratogenicity, Mutagenicity, and Carcinogenicity

Oral doses up to 300 mg/kg in mice, up to 200 mg/kg in rats, and up to 100 mg/kg in rabbits were not teratogenic.

Seven different in vitro and in vivo mutagenicity tests with oxprenolol were carried out using various concentrations: 25–2,025 μg/0.1 ml; 300, 580 μg/ml, or doses of 40, 120 mg/kg; 2 × 260, 520, 1,040 mg/kg; 42, 126 mg/kg. No signs of mutagenicity were observed.

In carcinogenicity studies, mice were treated for 180 days with approximately 8.3, 27, and 82 mg/kg daily in the feed. Supplementary studies in mice were carried out for 18 months with 15, 50, and 150 mg/kg of oxprenolol daily in the feed. Rats were treated for 180 days with 15, 50, and 150 mg/kg daily in the feed. Neither in mice nor in rats was evidence of a carcinogenic potential found.

Prescribing Notes – ®Trasicor (Oxprenolol)

Properties

®Trasicor is a nonselective beta-blocker exhibiting a judiciously balanced degree of intrinsic sympathomimetic activity. It is particularly suitable for the treatment of hypertension, angina pectoris, and sympathicotonic cardiovascular disorders. It also diminishes morbidity and mortality following myocardial infarction. Trasicor lowers elevated blood pressure both in the standing and in the supine position. Postural hypotension or disturbances in the electrolyte balance do not occur. In patients with angina pectoris, Trasicor reduces the frequency and severity of the attacks and increases physical working capacity. It exerts an antiarrhythmic effect by eliminating excessive catecholamine activity and by prolonging atrioventricular conduction time. The intrinsic sympathomimetic activity of Trasicor lessens its risk of provoking heart failure, bronchospasm, or peripheral circulatory disturbances.

Indications

Hypertension: as monotherapy or in combination with other antihypertensives, preferably with a diuretic (®Esidrex, ®Hygroton) and/or with a peripheral vasodilator (®Apresoline, ®Nepresol).

Angina pectoris: for long-term prophylactic use (nitroglycerin should if necessary be given to alleviate acute attacks).

For the reduction of morbidity and mortality after myocardial infarction (secondary prevention).

Disturbances of cardiac rhythm: especially supraventricular tachycardia, atrial fibrillation, and digitalis-induced arrhythmias; Trasicor is also indicated in ventricular tachycardia.

Functional sympathicotonic cardiovascular disorders: such as cardiac neurosis, hyperkinetic heart syndrome, and psychogenic (anxiety-induced) cardiovascular disorders.

Dosage and Administration

The tablets should be swallowed whole. Administering relatively high daily dosages in two divided doses serves to maintain good tolerability.

Hypertension: 160 mg daily, given either as a single dose in the morning or in two divided doses (morning and evening). If necessary, the dosage can be raised to 320–480 mg. When administering Trasicor as monotherapy, no advantage is gained by exceeding the maximum recommended dosages, since experience has shown that hardly any increase in the response can be achieved by this means. To enhance the therapeutic effect, it is advisable to resort to combined therapy.

Angina pectoris: 160 mg daily, given in 1–3 divided doses. If necessary, the dosage can be increased to 320–480 mg. In certain cases a daily dosage of 80 mg may suffice.

For the reduction of morbidity and mortality after myocardial infarction: 40 mg twice daily. The treatment should be initiated within the first few months (as soon as possible after hemodynamic stabilization has occurred following the acute event) and not interrupted without medical consultation.

Disturbances of cardiac rhythm and tachycardia: 40 mg 2–3 times daily orally. The daily dosage may later have to be individually adapted to the patient's requirements.

In the presence of arrhythmia and tachycardia, Trasicor can also be administered parenterally, provided heart rate, blood pressure, and ECG are monitored. For such treatment, the dry active substance contained in 1 ampoule (2 mg) should be dissolved in 5 ml of physiologic saline or sterile water for injection. The recommended initial dose is 2 mg, given slowly over 30 s, by intravenous injection. If no adequate response is obtained within 5 min, additional doses of 2 mg can be given at 5-min intervals. In persistent atrial arrhythmias, doses of up to a total of 16 mg may be required.

Functional sympathicotonic cardiovascular disorders: small daily doses of 40–80 mg are often sufficient.

Contraindications

These are: atrioventricular block of second or third degree, heart failure refractory to digitalis, marked bradycardia, and cardiogenic shock.

Precautions

Owing to the risk of bronchoconstriction, particular caution should be exercised when using Trasicor in patients with bronchial asthma (or with a history of bronchial asthma), chronic bronchitis, or emphysema. In such patients, treatment, given under surveillance, should be initiated with small doses which should then gradually be raised, until the optimum dosage has been reached. It is generally advisable in cases of this kind to prescribe the daily dosage in 3–4 divided doses. When treating patients with asthma, concomitant therapy with a beta-2-stimulant (e.g., terbutaline) should as a rule be administered. The dosage of bronchodilator medication should be readjusted when starting treatment with Trasicor.

Patients suffering from heart failure require adequate digitalization (supplemented, if necessary, by a diuretic) both before and during treatment with Trasicor. Trasicor does not interfere with the positive inotropic effect of digitalis. Special caution is required when administering beta-blockers intravenously. When performing routine measurements, patients' blood pressure and heart rate should be monitored. In exceptional cases, if pronounced bradycardia occurs, the dosage of Trasicor should be reduced or the preparation withdrawn.

Diabetic patients, especially those dependent on insulin, should be advised that treatment with beta-blockers may mask the symptoms of hypoglycemia. Since Trasicor may also affect carbohydrate metabolism, the dosage of hypoglycemic medication may have to be readjusted. Beta-blockers may also mask the signs and symptoms of a thyrotoxic crisis.

In patients with metabolic acidosis, particular caution should be observed because beta-blockade may impair the sympathetic nervous tone required in such cases to maintain vital functions.

Note

As with other beta-blockers, when discontinuing treatment with Trasicor, the drug should be withdrawn gradually over 7–10 days because abrupt interruption of the medication – particularly in patients with ischemic heart disease – may lead to an acute deterioration of the patient's condition.

When surgery is performed on patients under treatment with beta-blockers, the anesthetic selected should have as little negative inotropic activity as possible. The anesthetist should be informed in advance that the patient is receiving a beta-blocker. If Trasicor must be withdrawn before surgery, the dosage should be reduced gradually, and, if possible, the drug should be stopped at least 48 h before the induction of anesthesia.

Pregnancy and Lactation

During pregnancy, in the course of labor, and in nursing mothers, Trasicor should only be used provided due attention is paid to the possible effects, such as slowing of the heart rate, which its beta-blocking action may exert on the fetus, newborn infant, and breast-fed babies of mothers treated with the drug.

Adverse Effects

Occasionally, especially at the start of treatment, Trasicor – like other beta-blockers – may give rise to gastrointestinal upsets, dizziness, sleep disturbances, or exertional tiredness. These effects, however, are mild and seldom necessitate a dosage reduction. In rare cases hypersensitivity reactions (itching and reddening of the skin), feelings of coldness in the extremities, and thrombocytopenia have been reported. Provided the restrictions on the use of Trasicor are observed, severe bradycardia, heart failure, or bronchospasm are seldom encountered.

Interactions

Trasicor should not be given in combination with calcium antagonists of the verapamil type, because their concomitant use may result in bradycardia, hypotension, or even cardiac arrest.

Poisoning and Countermeasures

Overdosage may lead to pronounced hypotension and bradycardia. As a countermeasure, 1–2 mg atropine sulfate should be injected intravenously and, if this proves insufficient, pressor substances such as isoproterenol should be administered. Glucagon, at a dose of 1 mg, may also be given parenterally.

Other Preparations Containing Oxprenolol

To enable treatment for the various indications to be optimally adapted to the patient's individual requirements, Trasicor is available in several oral dosage strengths (40, 80, or 160 mg), in ampoules and also in sustained-release formulations (80 and 160 mg).

In countries where fixed drug combinations are in widespread use, combined preparations containing oxprenolol plus a diuretic and/or a vasodilator are available for the treatment of hypertension.

Because of stipulations laid down by the respective regulatory authorities, not all these dosage strengths and dosage forms have been introduced in every country. Information on the preparations available in a given country can be obtained from the local Ciba-Geigy organization.

References

1 Ahlquist, R.P.: A study of the adrenotropic receptors. Am. J. Physiol. *153:* 586 (1948).

2 Barnett, D.B.; Rugg, E.L.; Nahorski, S.R.: Direct evidence of two types of beta-adrenoceptor binding site in lung tissue. Nature *273:* 166 (1978).

3 Brechbühler, S.; Brunner, H.; Meier, M.; Orwin, J.; Rogg, H.: Oxprenolol; in Scriabine, Pharmacology of antihypertensive drugs, pp. 209–222 (Raven Press, New York 1980).

4 Brunner, H.; Hedwall, P.R.; Maier, R.; Meier, M.: Pharmacological aspects of oxprenolol. Post-grad. med. J., suppl., pp. 5–14 (1970).

5 Ciba-Geigy: Internal Reports of Pharmacologic Chemistry Department (unpublished).
6 Data on file (Ciba-Geigy Ltd., Basel).
7 Dawes, C.P.; Kendall, M.J.; Welling, P.G.: Bioavailability of conventional and slow release oxprenolol in fasted and nonfasted individuals. Br. J. clin. Pharmacol. *7:* 299 (1979).
8 Evans, G.H.; Nies, A.S.; Shand, D.G.: The disposition of propranolol. Decreased half-life and volume of distribution as a result of plasma binding in man, monkey, dog and rat. J. Pharmac. exp. Ther. *186:* 114 (1973).
9 Garteiz, D.A.: Metabolism of a beta-blocking drug, oxprenolol. J. Pharmac. exp. Ther. *179:* 354 (1971).
10 Goodman, L.S.; Gilman, A.: The pharmacological basis of therapeutics; 6th ed. (MacMillan, New York 1980).
11 Hellenbrecht, D.; Lemmer, B.; Wiethold, G.; Grobecker, H.: Measurement of hydrophobicity, surface activity, local anaesthesia, and myocardial conduction velocity as quantitative parameters of the nonspecific membrane affinity of nine beta-adrenergic blocking agents. Naunyn-Schmiedebergs Arch. exp. Path. Pharmak. *227:* 211 (1973).
12 Kendall, M.J.; Michard, M.; West, M.; John, V.A.; Ebbutt, A.F.: Factors influencing the absorption of oxprenolol: a pharmacokinetic study. Eur. J. Drug Metab. Pharmacokinet. *3:* 155 (1976).
13 Leeson, G.A.; Garteiz, D.A.; Knapp, W.C.; Wright, G.J.: Oxprenolol quantitation and metabolite identification (Abstract No. 3002). Fed. Proc. *32:* 747 (1977).
14 Mason, W.D.; Winer, N.: Pharmacokinetics of oxprenolol in normal subjects. Clin. Pharmacol. Ther. *20:* 401 (1976).
15 Meier, M.; Hedwall, P.R.; Imhof, P.; Wilhelm, M.; Brunner, H.: Untersuchungen mit den optischen Antipoden des adrenergischen Beta-Rezeptorenblockers 1-(*o*-allyloxyphenoxy)-3-(isopropyl-amino)-2-propanol. Arzneimittel-Forsch. *20:* 1890 (1970).
16 Nayler, W.G.; Chang, A.: Cellular pharmacology of beta-blocking drugs; in Burley, New perspectives in beta-blockade, pp. 41–71 (Ciba Laboratories, Horsham 1973).
17 Riess, W.; Brechbühler, S.; Theobald, W.: The pharmacokinetic characteristics of beta-receptor antagonists in man – similarities and differences of clinical relevance. Aust. N.Z. J. Med. *6:* suppl. 3, p. 4 (1976).
18 Riess, W.; Hürzeler, H.; Raschdorf, F.: The metabolites of oxprenolol (Trasicor®) in man. Xenobiotica *4:* 365 (1974).
19 Riess, W.; Rajagopalan, T.G.; Imhof, P.; Schmid, K.; Keberle, H.: Metabolic studies on oxprenolol in animals and man by means of radiotracer techniques and GLC analysis. Post-grad. med. J., suppl., p. 32 (1970).
20 Truelove, J.F.; Petten, G.R. van; Willes, R.F.: Action of several beta-adrenoceptor blocking drugs in the pregnant sheep and foetus. Br. J. Pharmacol. *47:* 161 (1973).
21 West, M.J.; Kendall, M.J.; Mitchard, M.; Faragher, E.B.: A comparison of slow release with conventional oxprenolol: plasma concentrations and clinical effects. Br. J. clin. Pharmacol. *3:* 439 (1976).

Jacob V. Aranda, Associate Professor and Director, Developmental Pharmacology, McGill University, Montreal, Que. (Canada)

Clinical Results

Stanley H. Taylor

Leeds, England

Introduction

The development of drugs capable of competitively blocking specific circulatory beta-adrenoceptors is a major therapeutic advance. Oxprenolol, one of the earliest drugs in this field, was, at the time of its introduction, the only nonselective beta-blocking drug with the additional pharmacologic property of intrinsic sympathomimetic activity, also referred to as partial agonist activity. Beta-blocking drugs, including oxprenolol, are useful both in the treatment and in the prevention of cardiovascular disease. It is, therefore, instructive to consider the role of the drug in both respects (fig. 1).

Oxprenolol in the Treatment of Cardiovascular Disorders

The beta-blockers were initially developed by Sir *James Black* for the treatment of angina pectoris, but the fortuitous discovery that they lowered blood pressure in angina patients led to their increasing use as antihypertensive agents. More recently, they were also found to be of distinct therapeutic value in a range of less sinister symptomatic syndromes. The indications for these drugs, including oxprenolol, may, therefore, be conveniently divided into those in which they play a major role and those in which their role is complementary to other treatments (table I).

Oxprenolol in Angina pectoris

The relief of exercise-inducing anginal pain in patients with coronary artery obstruction still provides the most dramatic vindication of the development of beta-blocking drugs. In this condition, they undoubtedly remain

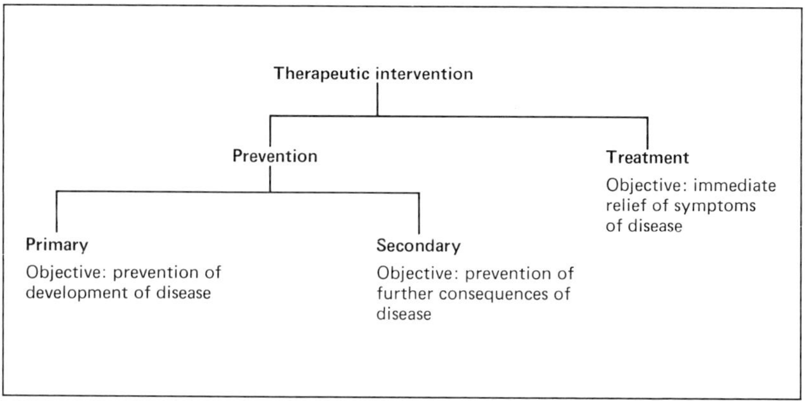

Fig. 1. Profile of therapeutic intervention.

Table I. Therapeutic indications for beta-adrenoceptor antagonists

Major	Minor
Hypertension	psychic stress
Coronary heart disease	anxiety states
Angina	thyrotoxicosis
Postmyocardial infarction	cardiomyopathy
Dysrhythmias	muscle tremor
	migraine

the treatment of choice. Oxprenolol extends the time walked before the onset of anginal pain in a predictable log-dose fashion (fig. 2). These effects are accompanied by similar attenuation of the degree of electrocardiographic S-T segment depression (fig. 3). The onset and duration of action of a single dose of oxprenolol is related to its rapid absorption and metabolic handling. Relief of exercise-induced angina pain is discernible within 30 min, reaches a peak between 1 and 2 h, and thereafter gradually declines (fig. 4). During chronic treatment, the degree to which anginal symptoms are relieved and the extent of improvement in the electrocardiogram are maintained; in this respect oxprenolol is the equal of other beta-adrenoceptor antagonists (fig. 5).

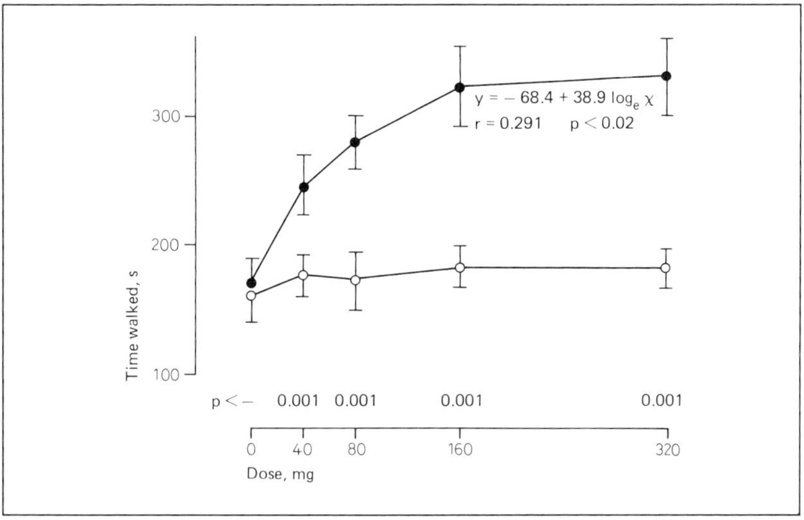

Fig. 2. Demonstration of the dose-response increase in walking time before the onset of anginal pain induced by oxprenolol in 16 patients with angina pectoris. ● = Oxprenolol; ○ = placebo [from ref. 42, with permission].

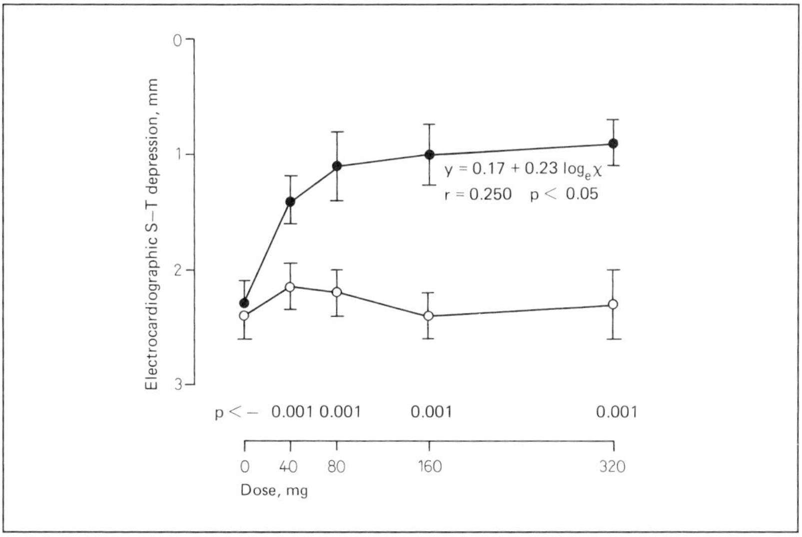

Fig. 3. Reduction of electrocardiographic S-T depression at the onset of exercise-induced anginal pain relative to the dose of oxprenolol in 16 patients with angina pectoris. ● = Oxprenolol; ○ = placebo.

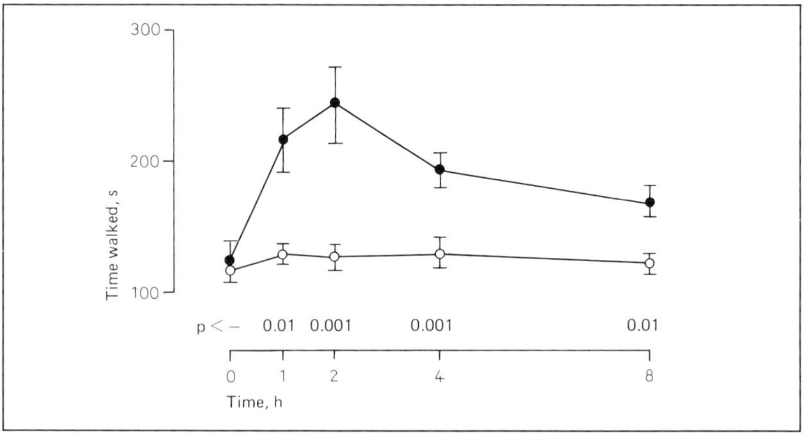

Fig. 4. Duration of action of a single oral dose of 160 mg oxprenolol on walking time before the onset of pain in 16 patients with angina pectoris. ● = Oxprenolol; ○ = placebo.

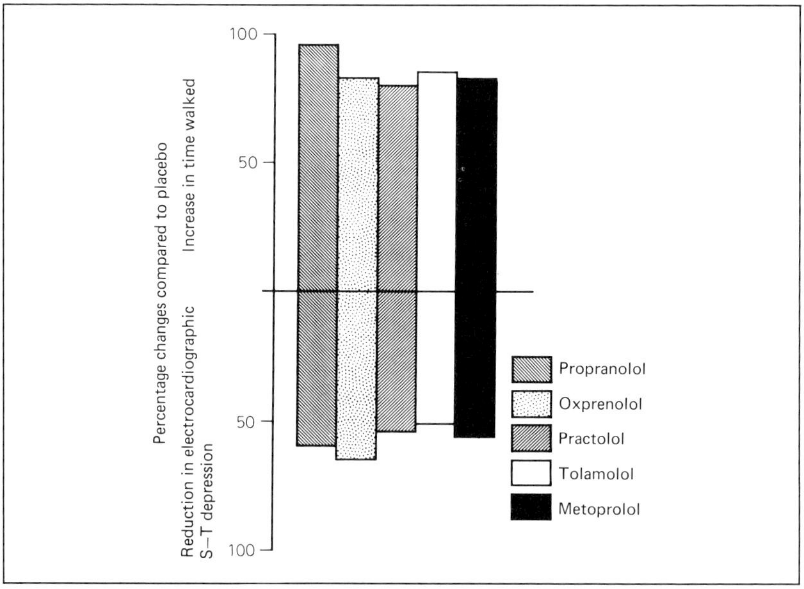

Fig. 5. Comparison of effects of beta-blocking drugs with different ancillary pharmacologic properties on time-to-angina and associated electrocardiographic changes during sustained treatment in 16 patients with angina pectoris. Results of a double-blind randomized cross-over study [from ref. 44, with permission].

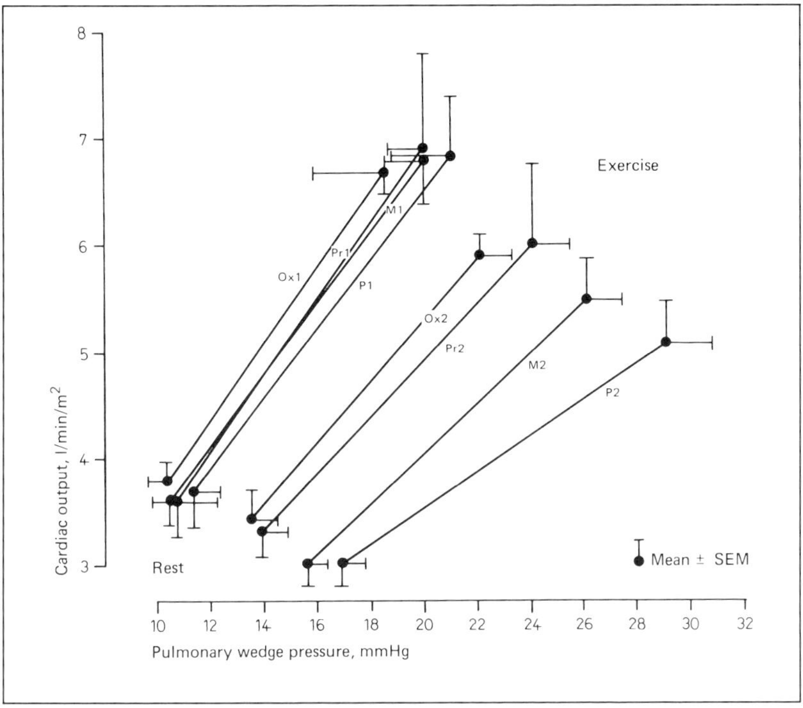

Fig. 6. Hemodynamic effects of four beta-adrenoceptor antagonists on the relation between left ventricular filling pressure output in 24 patients with stable coronary heart disease. Ox = Oxprenolol; P = propranolol; Pr = practolol; M = metoprolol. The numbers 1 and 2 relate to control and postdrug studies, respectively [from ref. 43, with permission].

The effects on left ventricular function of long-term treatment with oral oxprenolol of patients with angina pectoris is unknown. However, its immediate effects appear to be less deleterious to the pumping function of the left ventricle than are beta-blocking drugs without intrinsic sympathomimetic activity (fig. 6). In these patients, oxprenolol also induced less of an increase in peripheral vascular resistance, with the inference that there was less of an increase in left ventricular afterload and less peripheral vasoconstriction [43]. The efficacy of oxprenolol in the treatment of angina pectoris is, therefore, related both to its beta-blocking potency and to its intrinsic sympathomimetic activity (ISA).

Oxprenolol in the Treatment of Dysrhythmias

Ischemia of the myocardium frequently gives rise to a wide range of dysrhythmias. In exercise-induced angina pectoris, these usually present as ventricular ectopic beats, against which oxprenolol has been shown to be specifically effective [36].

Intravenous oxprenolol has also been shown to effectively abort many of the dysrhythmias that complicate acute myocardial infarction [38].

Oxprenolol in Hypertension

The mechanisms by which chronic blockade of beta-adrenoceptors lowers systemic arterial blood pressure are complex. However, the antihypertensive efficacy of the beta-blocking drugs is undoubted, and oxprenolol is no exception [6]. As would be expected from its specific beta-blocking activity, the immediate effects of its administration are on heart rate and systolic blood pressure which are reduced in a log-dose fashion during dynamic exercise (fig. 7). The onset and duration of these hemodynamic effects during exercise are related to its absorption and metabolic handling and follow a profile similar to that observed in angina. During chronic treatment, oxprenolol reduces heart rate as well as systolic and diastolic pressure at rest and suppresses the normal increase in heart rate and systolic pressure during walking, effects equal to those of other beta-blocking drugs (fig. 8). Thus, by lowering the resting blood pressure in hypertensive patients and preventing the potentially hazardous surges in systolic pressure and heart rate that occur in ambulant subjects during normal daily life, oxprenolol furnishes an efficacious antihypertensive prescription. This, together with the ability to suppress cardiac stimulation during psychic stress, affords a major therapeutic hope that oxprenolol will prevent the major cardiovascular complications of high blood pressure.

Minor Indications for Oxprenolol

Oxprenolol has been shown to be helpful in a number of conditions less sinister than coronary heart disease and hypertension. Psychic stress is often associated with marked stimulation of the cardiovascular system through the sympathoadrenal pathways [39]. In patients with declared cor-

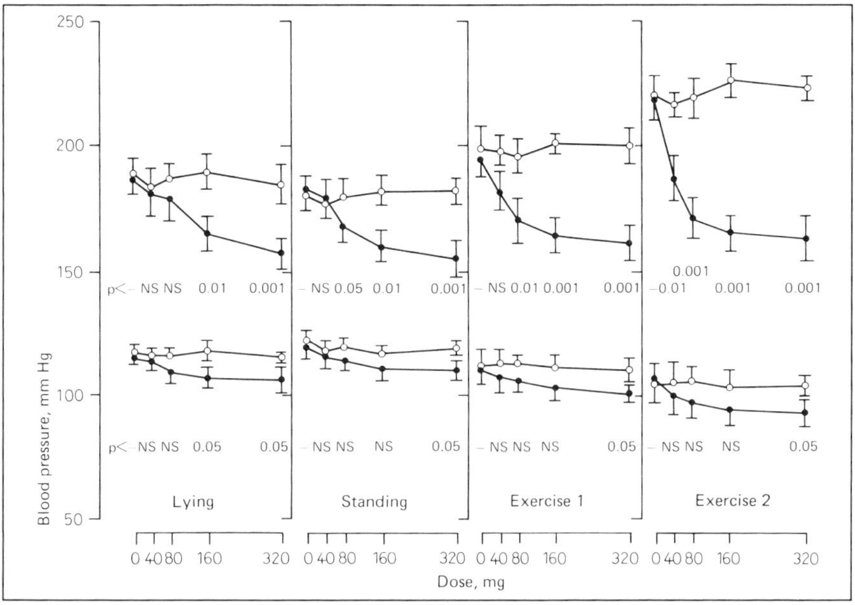

Fig. 7. Dose-response effects of oxprenolol 1 h after oral administration on the blood pressure lying and standing at rest and during two levels of treadmill walking in 25 hypertensive patients. ○ = Placebo; ● = oxprenolol.

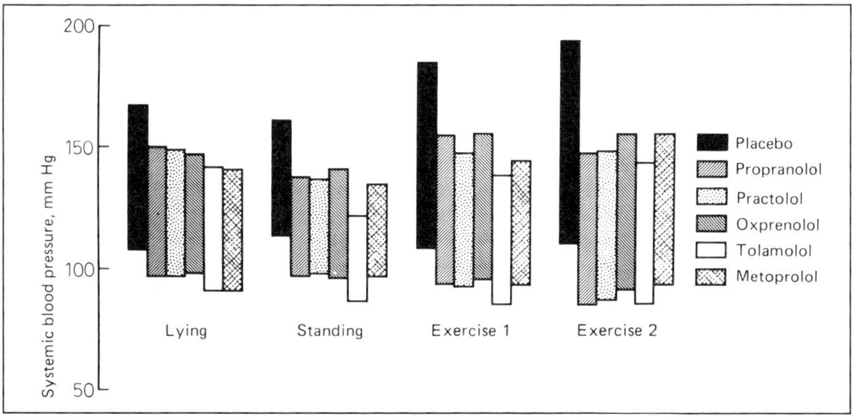

Fig. 8. Blood pressure after 8 weeks treatment (measured 1 h after oral dose). Comparative antihypertensive activity at rest and during two levels of treadmill walking of five beta-blocking drugs with different ancillary pharmacological properties in 25 hypertensive patients during sustained treatment [from ref. 5, with permission].

onary heart disease and in those with high blood pressure such stimulation may be hazardous. Oxprenolol was the first beta-blocking drug shown to effectively suppress such surges in psychosomatic stimulation [40]. Relatively small doses of the drug prevent the increases in sympathoadrenal stimulation of the cardiovascular system during motorcar driving, flying, television viewing, and during a range of other normal daily activities. The protection afforded to the ischemic myocardium has been demonstrated by the suppression of dysrhythmias in coronary-prone subjects during the stress of public speaking [35].

A major factor contributing to persistent symptoms in anxiety is the somatic awareness of sympathoadrenal stimulation of the heart. Somatic symptoms such as these may be readily blocked with small doses of oxprenolol, with outstanding benefit to the overall relief of this psychically engendered syndrome [12, 22].

The efficiency with which many testing activities are performed depends on the precise control of striated muscle function, e.g., playing music, playing bowls, and so on. Excessive sympathoadrenal circulation may be self-sustaining and counterproductive in these cases, and small doses of oxprenolol have been shown to improve performance of the task, often strikingly [14, 15, 32].

Cigarette smoking is associated with marked sympathoadrenal stimulation caused by stimulation of the vasomotor centers and the release of catecholamines from the adrenal medulla by the absorbed nicotine. Such repetitive stimulation of the cardiovascular system, together with the absorption of other noxious chemicals, may prove hazardous to coronary-prone or hypertensive patients. In normal subjects and in patients with ischemic heart disease oxprenolol reduced catecholamine-induced cardiac stimulation and the associated rise in plasma concentrations of free fatty acids induced by cigarette smoking (fig. 9) [4, 41].

A major component of the common social syndrome referred to as 'examination nerves' is the awareness of somatic manifestations of sympathoadrenal stimulation, e.g., palpitations, finger tremors, and so on. These symptoms of anxiety are reduced by small doses of oxprenolol, without any reduction in intellectual performance [17].

Oxprenolol possesses potent beta-blocking activity, and its therapeutic efficacy in clinical practice has been noted repeatedly. In contrast, there are few topics in cardiovascular medicine that have caused such debate as the therapeutic role of its intrinsic sympathomimetic activity (ISA). The theoretical therapeutic potential of ISA is easy to understand, but its impact in

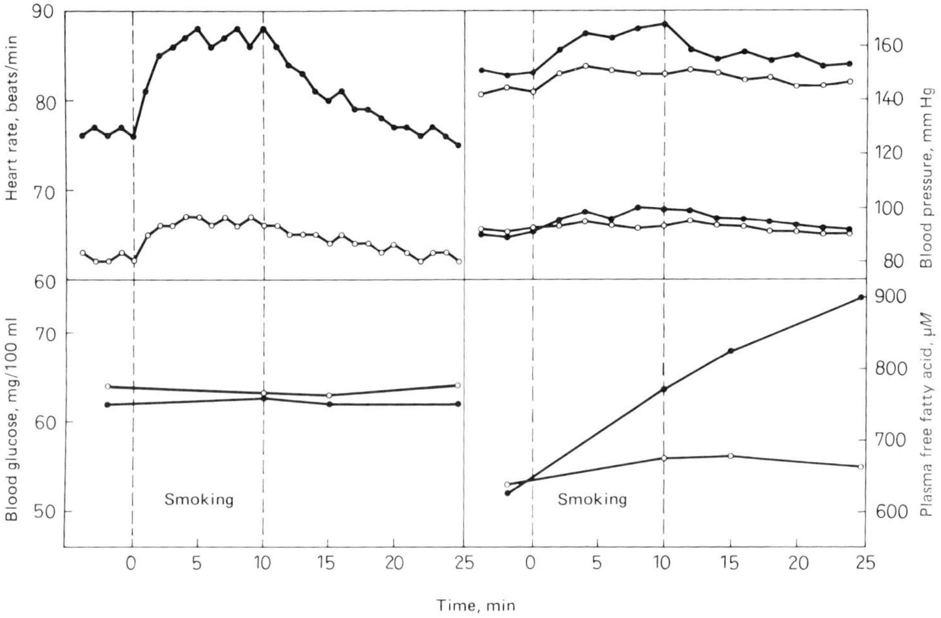

Fig. 9. Circulatory and metabolic effects of cigarette smoking in 24 patients with ischemic heart disease before and 1 h after 40 mg oral oxprenolol. ● = After placebo; ○ = after oxprenolol [from ref. 42, with permission].

clinical practice is more subtle and always subordinate to the prime beta-blocking activity of the drug. It is relevant, therefore, to review the evidence that ISA may offer additional advantages in the treatment of patients, when a beta-blocking drug is being considered for use. This particularly pertains to oxprenolol, as its moderate ISA is the specific pharmacologic property that sets this drug apart from other beta-blocking drugs.

Pharmacology of ISA

How can a molecule of oxprenolol block and, to a lesser extent, stimulate a beta-adrenoceptor at the same time? Intrinsic sympathomimetic activity is the property of the catecholamine-like molecular structure of the drug. A pure agonist, such as isoprenaline, has a molecular structure optimal for maximum stimulation of a beta-adrenoceptor. The molecular structure of oxprenolol is optimal for blocking, but less than optimal for stimulating beta-receptors. Thus, when oxprenolol combines with a beta-receptor, its excess catecholamine cannot bind to that receptor (its beta-blocking component); at the same time the catecholamine-like molecular configuration of oxprenolol results in partial stimulation of the same receptor (its intrinsic sympathomimetic activity, ISA). It also follows that beta-blocking drugs with ISA may have a similar blocking, but different stimulating facilities for beta-adrenoceptors.

Pharmacodynamic Demonstration of ISA

The relative degree of ISA in a beta-blocking drug may be demonstrated, if other sympathoadrenal influences are excluded, e.g., in the isolated atria of the cat (fig. 10). The positive stimulation induced by ISA may also be demonstrated on the contractile force developed in isolated strips of heart muscle or in the heart of the reserpinized (i.e., catecholamine-depleted) conscious animal.

The influence of ISA on the beta-blocking effect of a drug may clearly be seen in the smooth muscle of peripheral vessels [5, 33]. The contractile tone of peripheral arteriolar resistance vessels is the result of competing influences of vasoconstrictor alpha-1-adrenoceptors and vasodilator beta-2-adrenoceptors. Thus, ISA has little influence on vascular resistance in regions with predominantly alpha-1 representation – e.g., skin and kidney. But in regions where beta-2-adrenoceptors predominate – e.g., mesentery and striated muscles –, beta-blocking drugs with ISA result in less increase in vascular resistance than do those without this property.

It is now apparent that the effects of ISA are not the same in all tissues. The relaxing effects of ISA on the smooth muscle of arteriolar resistance vessels through stimulation of beta-2-adrenoceptors is far greater than the effect of stimulation of the same receptors in the bronchi or beta-1-adrenoceptors in the heart (fig. 11). The degree of ISA exerted by a beta-blocking drug is directly related to the dose used, but the net effect is inversely related to the level of prevailing sympathetic tone. For example, the pharmacodynamic effects of ISA in a beta-blocking drug are maximal during periods of low sympathetic drive, e.g., at rest or during sleep. Conversely, the influence of ISA is difficult to discern during states of high sympathetic drive – e.g., maximum exercise –, where the direct effects of beta-blockade predominate.

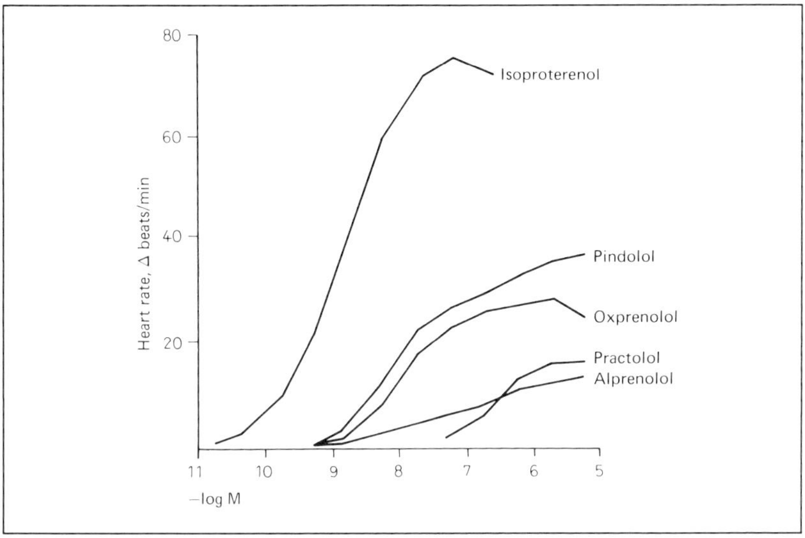

Fig. 10. Positive chronotropic effects of four beta-blocking drugs with intrinsic sympathomimetic activity in the isolated right atrium of the cat [from ref. 16, with permission].

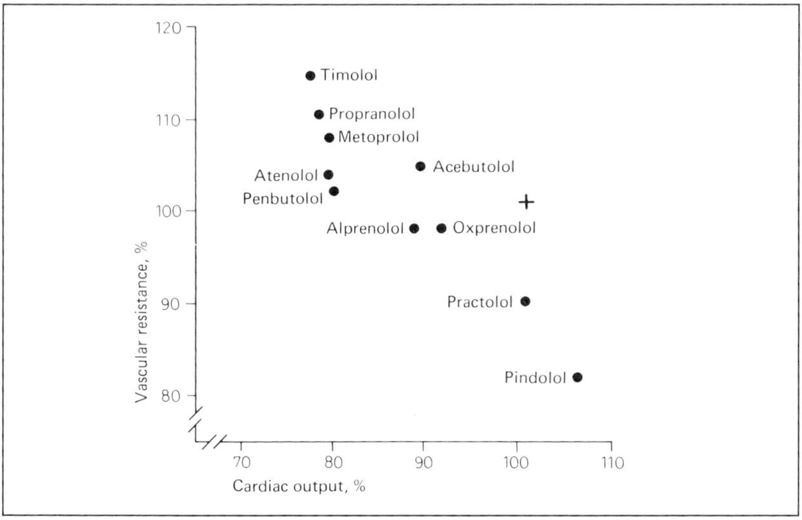

Fig. 11. Hemodynamic effects of beta-adrenoceptor blocking drugs with different degrees of ISA in 396 hypertensive patients [abstracted from ref. 19]. The black cross indicates the pretreatment values.

Clinical Potential of ISA

The experimental basis for the pharmacodynamic demonstration of ISA in a beta-blocking drug is now firmly established. Can this property be discerned in the far more complex reflexly intact animal or man, particularly in the presence of concurrent beta-blockade?

The net pharmacologic activity of a beta-blocking drug with ISA should be reflected in less negative chronotropic activity, less negative inotropic activity, less peripheral vasoconstriction, and less bronchoconstriction. On theoretical grounds, it is to be expected that stimulation of the sinus node and A-V conduction system during periods of low sympathetic activity may reduce the risk of undesirable bradycardia and heart block. Direct stimulation of the myocardium by ISA and a reduction in left ventricular afterload due to the reduced peripheral vascular resistance could also be expected to result in less depression of left ventricular pumping function, particularly in the compromised heart. Stimulation of beta-2-bronchodilator receptors could also be expected to offset some of the bronchoconstrictor effects of beta-blockade, particularly during exercise. Taken together, it is possible that the less depression in cardiac pumping function and the less bronchoconstriction afforded by a beta-blocking drug with ISA would result in less depression of exercise capacity than observed with beta-blockers that do not have this ancillary pharmacologic property. Beta-blocking drugs with ISA should also cause less peripheral vasoconstriction than do those without this property. Whether such clearly defined potential attributes are translated into discernible therapeutic benefits has not been proven as yet.

Therapeutic Impact of ISA

It is instructive to examine the evidence in man, which may point to the clinical advantage of beta-blockade and concurrent intrinsic sympathomimetic activity, such as that possessed by oxprenolol.

Effects on Heart Rate

Beta-blocking drugs with ISA result in less reduction in the resting heart rate than do drugs without this property. These effects are most marked at rest. Thus, the circadian rhythm of the heart is changed in that the profound reduction during sleep is countered by ISA, while the tachycardia associated with ambulant activity is blocked by the beta-blocking component [10]. In this regard, beta-blocking drugs with ISA differ markedly from those without this property.

Left Ventricular Function

Beta-blockade results in depression of left ventricular pumping activity for three hemodynamic reasons: (1) left ventricular myocardial contractility is reduced; (2) heart rate is reduced, and (3) left ventricular afterload is increased due to blockade of peripheral vasodilator beta-2-adrenoceptors and reflex alpha-1-mediated vasoconstriction. ISA in a beta-blocking drug can be expected to offset each of these potential deleterious effects on the pumping function of the heart. The result is that beta-blocking drugs with ISA result in substantially less depression of ventricular pumping function than do those without this property, not only at rest but also during exercise [29, 43].

Peripheral Vascular Resistance

Beta-blocking drugs increase the systemic vascular resistance directly by blockade of vasodilator beta-2-adrenoceptors in arteriolar resistance vessels and indirectly by reflex vasoconstriction mediated through alpha-1-adrenoceptors secondary to the depression in left ventricular pumping activity. In both circumstances beta-blocking drugs with ISA do not increase the systemic vascular resistance as much as those without this subsidiary pharmacological property (fig. 12). Both finger (fig. 13) and forearm muscle (fig. 14) blood flows are also less reduced by beta-blocking drugs with ISA than by those without this property, at least at rest.

Bronchoconstriction

Beta-blockade increases airway resistance by blocking beta-2-adrenoceptors responsible for bronchial muscle relaxation. The effects of ISA are to offset the bronchoconstrictor effects of beta-blockade by stimulating bronchial relaxation. Drugs with a significant degree of ISA induce a lesser increase in airway resistance than do drugs without this subsidiary pharmacologic property, particularly during exercise (fig. 15) [7, 26].

Exercise Capacity

The cardiorespiratory and striated muscle elements that contribute to exercise tolerance are complex. Beta-blockade reduces exercise capacity by reducing perfusion to striated muscles, thus inducing precocious fatigue.

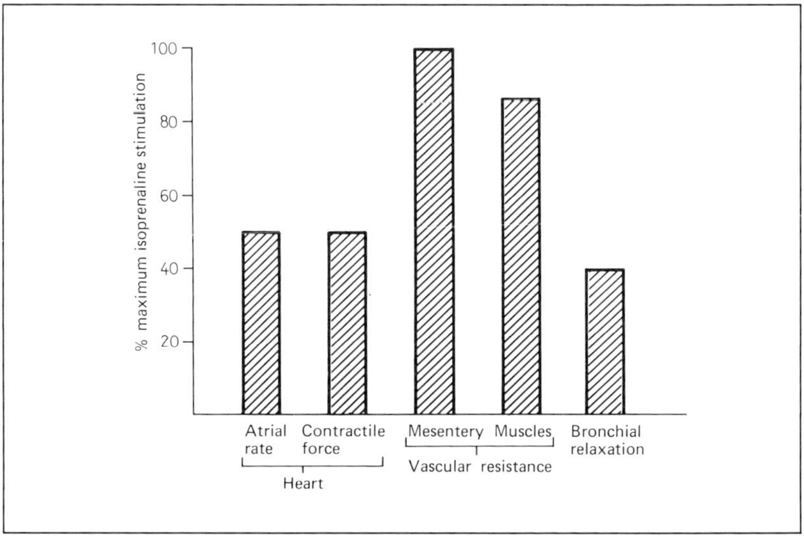

Fig. 12. Comparison of the maximum effects achieved by intrinsic sympathomimetic activity in different tissues compared to that achieved by isoprenaline.

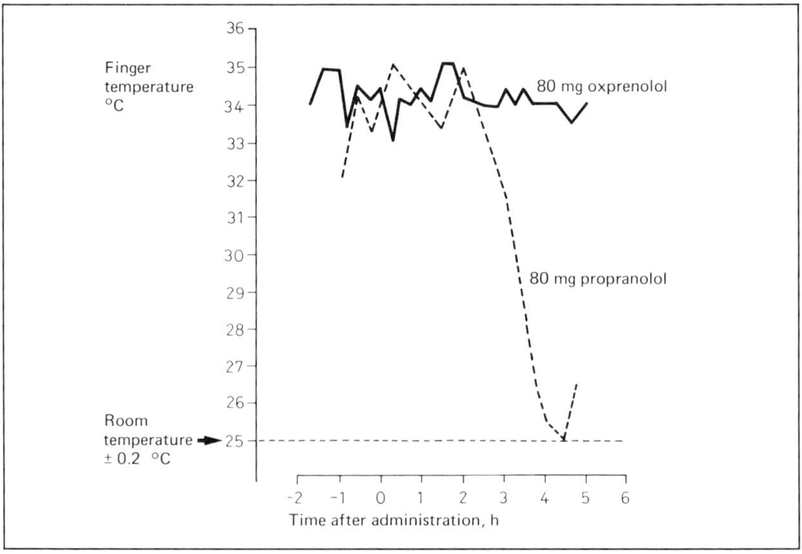

Fig. 13. Finger temperature following single oral doses of either propranolol or oxprenolol on separate occasions in a hypertensive patient [from ref. 30, with permission].

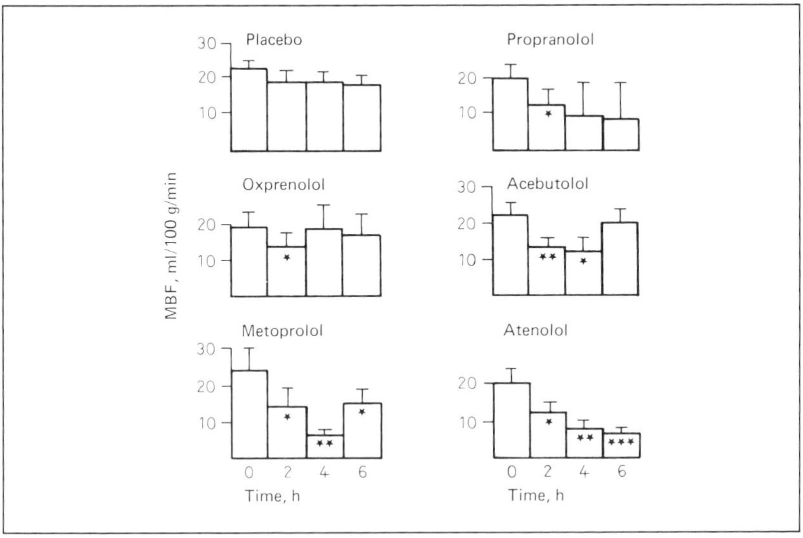

Fig. 14. Average exercise muscle blood flow (MBF) immediately before and 1, 2, 4 and 6 h after doses of drugs. p values express difference from 0 for each drug. * $p < 0.05$; ** $p < 0.005$; *** $p < 0.001$ [from ref. 33, with permission].

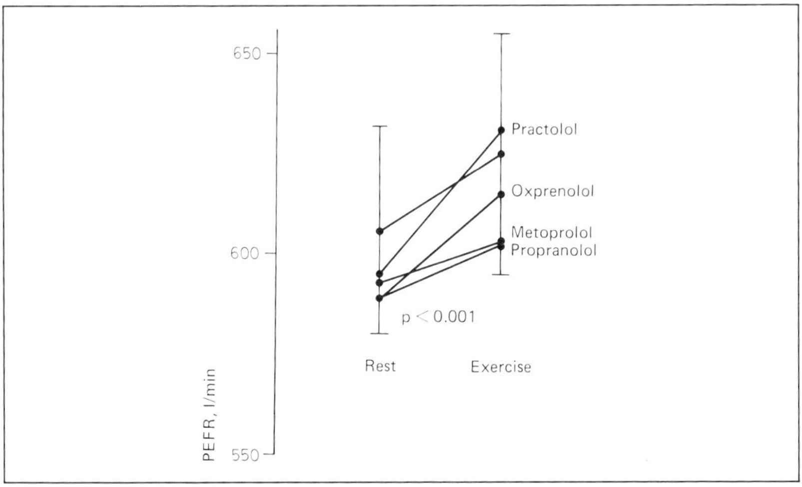

Fig. 15. Influence on peak expiratory flow rate (PEFR) of beta-blocking drugs with different ancillary pharmacologic properties at rest and during upright exercise in 6 normal subjects [from ref. 7, with permission].

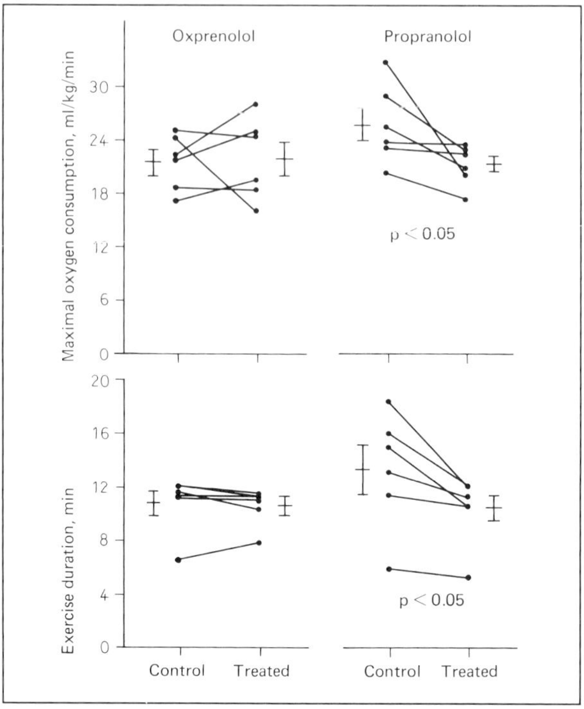

Fig. 16. Influence of ISA on exercise tolerance. Comparison of the effect of chronic treatment with oxprenolol or propranolol in hypertensive patients [from ref. 11, with permission].

The increase in pulmonary venous pressure and airway resistance also furnishes significant respiratory components in limiting the increased exercise capacity induced by beta-blockade. Each of these pharmacodynamic effects of beta-blockade alone are countered to a varying extent by ISA. Despite the complexity and difficulties of measuring exercise performance in patients, there are measurable indications that drugs with ISA depress exercise capacity less than those without this property (fig. 16) [11].

Blood Flow, Metabolism, and Function of the Ischemic Myocardium

The ischemic myocardium is particularly sensitive to the influence of sympathetic stimulation and its blockade. Thus, the overriding effects of a beta-blocking drug, with or without other ancillary pharmacologic properties, are due to its beta-blocking potency. There is some evidence that ISA may be important in protecting the ischemic myocardium, over and above that associated with blockade of myocardial oxygen-wasting sympathetic stimulation. Beta-blocking drugs with ISA appear to benefit the ischemic zone blood flow more than those without this property [20]. ISA also appears to prevent the lactate excretion that results when beta-blocking drugs without ISA are given [21]. This may explain why ISA appears to enhance the return to aerobic metabolism and functional recovery in transiently ischemic heart muscle [20]. It must be emphasized, however, that ISA plays a purely subordinate role to beta-blockade in this acute pathophysiologic situation.

Withdrawal Phenomenon

In patients with coronary heart disease the abrupt withdrawal of beta-blocking drugs may result in a resurgence in anginal pain, myocardial infarction, or sudden death [1, 8, 24, 25, 28, 31], related to the increased numbers or increased sensitivity of cardiac beta-receptors during sustained treatment with these drugs. It may be measured as an increase in the sensitivity of the heart rate to infused isoprenaline and an increase in resting heart rate for some days after these drugs are withdrawn. The possession of ISA by a beta-blocking drug appears to preclude these potentially hazardous phenomena [27]. This is particularly true of oxprenolol; no beta-adrenoceptor hypersensitivity was demonstrated after its abrupt withdrawal following long-term treatment in hypertension [2].

Blood Lipids

Beta-blocking drugs can influence the blood lipid level in three different ways: (1) sympathetic stimulation leads to the release of nonesterified fatty acids from activation of beta-1-adrenoceptors in adipose tissue; (2) high concentrations of plasma free fatty acids are potentially deleterious to the ischemic myocardium and, by overloading its aerobic metabolic capabilities, may induce life-threatening dysrhythmias, and (3) all beta-blocking drugs reduce the mobilization of these fatty acids, and ISA appears to have no direct influence in this regard.

ISA also has little or no discernible effect on plasma concentrations of triglycerides. However, it does play a potentially important role in regulating plasma concentrations of lipoprotein fractions carrying cholesterol. Sustained treatment with beta-blocking drugs without ISA reduces this ratio, due to an increase in low-density lipoprotein fractions [9, 13, 18, 32, 34, 35, 37]. In contrast, drugs with ISA appear to cause either no change in the high-density/low-density lipoprotein cholesterol ratio or an increased ratio [3, 13]. Epidemiologic studies have implicated the high-density/low-density lipoprotein cholesterol ratio as a potential marker of precocious atherogenesis [23]. Thus, the possession of ISA by a beta-blocking drug may be potentially advantageous in this regard, when long-term treatment of patients predisposed to coronary or cerebral arterial disease is considered.

Oxprenolol and ISA

Oxprenolol is first and foremost a potent beta-blocking drug and possesses the ancillary pharmacologic property of ISA which is entirely subsidiary to its beta-blocking activity, both from the pharmacodynamic aspect and its therapeutic importance. The pharmacodynamic profile of beta-blockers with ISA is clinically attractive. For example, the beta-blocking component of oxprenolol prevents the surges in sympathetic activity that are potentially deleterious to the heart and circulation; it suppresses these surges in a dose-response fashion. In contrast, ISA provides for background stimulation of beta-adrenoceptors, an effect that is also dose related. This combination of pharmacodynamic properties in oxprenolol can be expected to attenuate excessive sympathetic stimulation of the heart, while, at the same time, protecting the myocardium from the excessive withdrawal of all sympathomimetic support. In cases in which beta-blockade is judged to be therapeutically advantageous, the additional property of ISA is frequently an advantage and rarely, in this author's opinion, a disadvantage.

References

1 Alderman, E.L.; Coltart, D.J.; Wettach, G.E.; Harrison, D.C.: Coronary artery syndromes after sudden propranolol withdrawal. Ann. intern. Med. *81:* 625–627 (1974).

2 Bolli, P.; Fritz, R.B.; Raeder, E.A.; Amann, F.W.; Meier, M.; Rogg, H.; Burckhardt, D.: Lack of beta-adrenoceptor hypersensitivity after abrupt withdrawal of long-term therapy with oxprenolol. Circulation *64:* 1130–1134 (1981).

3 Bolli, P.; Stähelin, H.B.; Van Brummelen, P.; Kiowski, W.; Bühler, F.R.: Effect on plasma lipid fractions of long-term antihypertensive therapy with slow oxprenolol; in Burley, Birdwood, The clinical impact of beta-adrenoceptor blockade. Proc. Int. Symp., Berlin, pp. 239–247 (Ciba, Horsham 1980).

4 Carruthers, M.: Modification of the noradrenaline related effects of smoking by beta-blockade. Psychol. Med. *6:* 251 (1976).

5 Clark, B.J.; Menninger, K.; Bertholet, A.: Pindolol – the pharmacology of a partial agonist. Br. J. clin. Pharmacol. *13:* 149S–158S (1982).

6 Davidson, C.; Thadani, U.; Singleton, W.; Taylor, S.H.: Comparison of antihypertensive activity of beta-blocking drugs during chronic treatment. Br. med. J. *ii:* 1–8 (1976).
7 Davidson, C.; Kusail, A.A.; Taylor, S.H.: Comparative effects of beta-adrenoceptor antagonists on airways resistance at rest and during exercise in normal subjects. Br. J. clin. Pharmacol. *4:* 636P–637P (1977).
8 Diaz, R.G.; Somberg, J.C.; Freeman, E.; Levitt, B.: Withdrawal of propranolol and myocardial infarction. Lancet *i:* 1068 (1973).
9 England, J.D.F.; Simons, L.A.; Gibson, J.C.; Carlton, M.: The effects of metoprolol and atenolol on plasma high-density lipoprotein levels in man. Clin. exp. Pharmacol. Physiol. *7:* 329–333 (1980).
10 Fitscha, P.; Tiso, B.; Meisner, W.; Spitzer, D.: The effect of intrinsic sympathomimetic activity of beta-adrenoceptor blockers on circadian heart rate. Br. J. clin. Pharmacol. *13:* 211S–215S (1982).
11 Franciosa, J.A.; Johnson, S.M.; Tobian, L.J.: Exercise performance in mildly hypertensive patients. Impairment by propranolol but not oxprenolol. Chest *78:* 291–299 (1980).
12 Hawkings, J.R.: In a therapeutic approach to the psyche via the beta-adrenoceptor system. Proc. Symp. 6th Congr. of Psychiatry, Honolulu 1977.
13 Helgeland, A.; Hjermann, I.; Leren, P.; Enger, S.; Holme, I.: High-density lipoprotein cholesterol and anti-hypertensive drugs: the Oslo Study. Br. med. J. *ii:* 403 (1978).
14 James, I.M.; Pearson, R.M.; Griffith, D.N.W.; Newbury, P.: Effect of oxprenolol on stage-fright in musicians. Lancet *ii:* 952–954 (1977).
15 James, I.M.; Pearson, R.M.; Griffith, D.N.W.; Newbury, P.; Taylor, S.H.: The effect of oxprenolol on stress-induced disturbances of performance. Proc. R. Soc. Med. *70:* suppl. 11, p. 34 (1977).
16 Kauman, A.J.; Blink, J.R.: Beta-adrenoceptor blocking agents as partial agonists in isolated heart muscle: dissociation of stimulation and blockade. Arch. Pharmacol. *311:* 237–248 (1980).
17 Krishnan, G.: Oxprenolol in the treatment of examination nerves. Scott. med. J. *20:* 288–289 (1975).
18 Lehtonen, A.; Viikari, J.: Long-term effect of sotalol on plasma lipids. Clin. Sci. *57:* 405S–407S (1979).
19 Man In't Veld, A.J.; Schalekamp, M.A.D.H.: How intrinsic sympathomimetic activity modulates the haemodynamic responses to beta-adrenoceptor antagonists. A clue to the nature of their antihypertensive mechanism. Br. J. clin. Pharmacol. *13:* 245S–257S (1982).
20 Manning, A.S.; Keogh, J.M.; Shattock, M.J.; Coltart, D.J.; Hearse, D.J.: Long-term beta-blockade: prolonged protective action on the ischaemic myocardium. Cardiovasc. Res. *15:* 462–467 (1981).
21 Marshall, R.J.; Parratt, J.R.: A comparative study of beta-adrenoceptor blocking agents on blood flow and metabolism in the acutely ischaemic myocardium. Proc. R. Soc. Med. *70:* suppl. 11, pp. 62–68 (1977).
22 Michael, J.: A placebo-controlled double-blind trial of oxprenolol versus diazepam in the treatment of anxiety and stress; in Kielholz, Siegenthaler, Taggart, Zanchetti, Psychosomatic cardiovascular disorders – when and how to treat?, pp. 191–196 (Huber, Bern 1981).

23 Miller, G.J.; Miller, N.E.: Plasma-high-density-lipoprotein concentration and development of ischaemic heart disease. Lancet *i:* 16–19 (1975).
24 Miller, R.R.; Olson, H.G.; Amsterdam, E.A.; Mason, D.T.: Propranolol withdrawal rebound phenomenon: exacerbation of coronary events after abrupt cessation of antianginal therapy. New Engl. J. Med. *293:* 416–418 (1975).
25 Nattel, S.; Rangno, R.E.; Van Loon, G.: Mechanism of propranolol withdrawal phenomena. Circulation *59:* 1158–1164 (1979).
26 Oh, V.M.S.; Kaye, C.M.; Warrington, S.J.; Taylor, E.A.; Wadsworth, J.: Studies of cardioselectivity and partial agonist activity in beta-adrenoceptor blockade comparing effects on heart rate and peak expiratory flow rate during exercise. Br. J. clin. Pharmacol. *5:* 107–120 (1978).
27 Prichard, B.N.C.; Walden, R.J.: The syndrome associated with the withdrawal of beta-adrenergic receptor blocking drugs. Br. J. clin. Pharmacol. *13:* 337S–343S (1982).
28 Rangno, R.E.; Langlois, S.: Comparison of withdrawal phenomena after propranolol, metoprolol and pindolol. Br. J. clin. Pharmacol. *13:* 345S–351S (1982).
29 Reale, A.; Nigri, A.; Gioffre, P.A.; Motolese, M.: Acute influence of different beta-blocking agents upon left heart haemodynamics at rest and during exercise in patients with coronary artery disease. Eur. J. Cardiol. *9:* 101–109 (1979).
30 Roberts, C.J.C.; Marshall, A.J.; Barritt, D.W.: A study of cold extremities in patients taking beta-blocking drugs; in Judd, Topics in cardiovascular disease. Proc. Int. Symp., pp. 179–186 (Ciba, Horsham 1976).
31 Shiroff, R.A.; Mathis, J.; Zelis, R.; Schneck, D.W.; Babb, J.D.; Leaman, D.M.; Hayes, A.H.: Propranolol rebound – a retrospective study. Am. J. Cardiol. *41:* 778–780 (1978).
32 Siitonen, L.; Janne, J.: Effect of beta-blocking during bowling competitions. Ann. clin. Res. *8:* 393–398 (1976).
33 Smith, R.S.; Warren, D.J.: Effect of acute oral beta-adrenergic blockade on muscle blood flow in man. Cardiovasc. Res. *16:* 205–208 (1982).
34 Streja, D.; Mymin, D.: Effect of propranolol on HDL cholesterol concentrations. Br. med. J. *ii:* 1495 (1978).
35 Taggart, P.; Carruthers, M.; Somerville, W.: Electrocardiogram, plasma catecholamines and lipids and their modification by oxprenolol when speaking before an audience. Lancet *ii:* 341–346 (1973).
36 Taggart, P.; Carruthers, M.: Emotional stress-induced arrhythmias. Proc. R. Soc. Med. *70:* suppl. 11, pp. 41–43 (1977).
37 Tanaka, N.; Sakaguchi, S.; Oshige, K.; Niimura, T.; Kanehisa, T.: Effect of chronic administration of propranolol on lipoprotein composition. Metabolism *25:* 1071–1075 (1976).
38 Taylor, S.H.; Burley, D.M.: Beta-adrenoceptor blocking drugs in postmyocardial infarction dysrhythmias. Proc. R. Soc. Med. *70:* suppl. 11, pp. 11–19 (1977).
39 Taylor, S.H.: Stress, hypertension and ischaemic heart disease; in Kielholz, Siegenthaler, Taggart, Zanchetti, Psychosomatic cardiovascular disorders – when and how to treat?, pp. 120–137 (Huber, Bern 1981).
40 Taylor, S.H.; Meeran, M.K.: The cardiovascular response to some environmental stresses and their modification by oxprenolol; in Burley, New perspectives in beta-blockade. Int. Symp., Aarhus, pp. 293–306 (Ciba, Horsham 1973).

41 Taylor, S.H.; Pearson, M.C.; Myint, S.: Circulatory and metabolic effects of smoking cigarettes with and without tobacco substitute and their modulation by beta-receptor blockade. Q. Jl Med. *43:* 617 (1976).
42 Taylor, S.H.; Thadani, U.; Watt, S.J.; Goldstraw, P.W.; Hess, H.; Riess, W.: Studies with slow-release oxprenolol. II. Acute and chronic administration to patients with exercise-induced angina pectoris; in Judd, Topics in cardiovascular disease. Proc. Int. Symp., Basel, pp. 131–138 (Ciba, Horsham 1977).
43 Taylor, S.H.; Silke, B.; Lee, P.S.: Intravenous beta-blockade in coronary heart disease. New Engl. J. Med. *306:* 631–635 (1982).
44 Thadani, U.; Davidson, C.; Singleton, W.; Taylor, S.H.: Comparison of the immediate effects of five beta-receptor antagonists with different ancillary properties in angina pectoris. Am. J. Cardiol. *41:* 415 (1978).

S.H. Taylor, University Department of Cardiovascular Studies and Department of Medical Cardiology, The General Infirmary, Leeds (England)

Therapeutic Outlook

Oxprenolol in the Primary and Secondary Prevention of Coronary Heart Disease

Stanley H. Taylor

Leeds, England

Introduction

Coronary heart disease continues to remain a major health problem. Many risk factors have been shown to be associated with its precocious development (table I). These primary risk factors, some immutable and others susceptible to correction, exert an overriding influence on the development of the syndrome. However, once myocardial damage has occurred, the risk profile determining further prognosis is radically changed, and there is a steeply rising incidence of recurrent myocardial infarction and sudden cardiac death. Thus, the ultimate aim in any community health program devoted to the eradication of coronary heart disease must be directed to primary prevention, i.e., the interruption, delay, or reversal of pathologic processes responsible for the clinical presentation of the disease.

Prophylactic Treatment of Hypertension

Of the modifiable risk factors susceptible to therapeutic intervention, high blood pressure is by far the most important. The risk of developing a cardiovascular catastrophe is directly and independently related to the height of the blood pressure, particularly systolic blood pressure, in both sexes and particularly in middle and late life [35]. This predictable hazard is aggravated by many other biologic factors, e.g., hyperlipidemia, glucose intolerance, obesity, and others, by the personality type/behavior pattern of the individual, and by their personal habits, e.g., cigarette smoking, lack of exercise, and so on.

Pathophysiological Considerations for Antihypertensive Treatment

The coronary and cerebral arteries open directly off the aorta through relatively short muscular arteries and thus are little protected against the high-energy pressure waves generated by systolic contraction of the hypertrophied left ventricle. Mechanical trauma to the arterial wall is not only a function of the average pressure inside the artery, but it is also closely related to the energy imparted by the pressure wave (fig. 1). Increased amplitude of the pressure pulse in the hypertensive patient undoubtedly contributes to precocious arterial trauma. The period of the pressure wave is of much greater importance in the production of arterial damage than is its amplitude (fig. 2). The height of systolic blood pressure – and thus the amplitude of the pulse wave – and its period are all direct functions of the contractile behavior of the left ventricle. The frequency with which such pressure pulses are generated, i.e., the heart rate, is a direct function of the sinus node. Thus, sympathetic stimulation of beta-adrenoceptors in the left ventricle and the right atrium plays a major role in determining potential physical hazards to major vital arteries.

During normal daily life the blood pressure varies widely (fig. 3). Thus, the aim of antihypertensive treatment is most logically directed not only toward reducing the basal level, but also toward attenuating the surges in pressure. Beta-blocking drugs, including oxprenolol, are outstandingly efficacious in reducing the resting blood pressure (see figure 7, chapter 'Clinical Results'). They are also unique among non-beta-blocker antihypertensive drugs in reducing the surges in blood pressure and heart rate associated with ambulant activity (fig. 4), psychic stress, and cigarette smoking (see

Table I. Risk factors predisposing to coronary heart disease

Immutable	Possibly modifiable	Modifiable
Age	personality	blood pressure
Sex		smoking habits
Family history		occupation
		eating habits
		drinking habits
		exercise habits

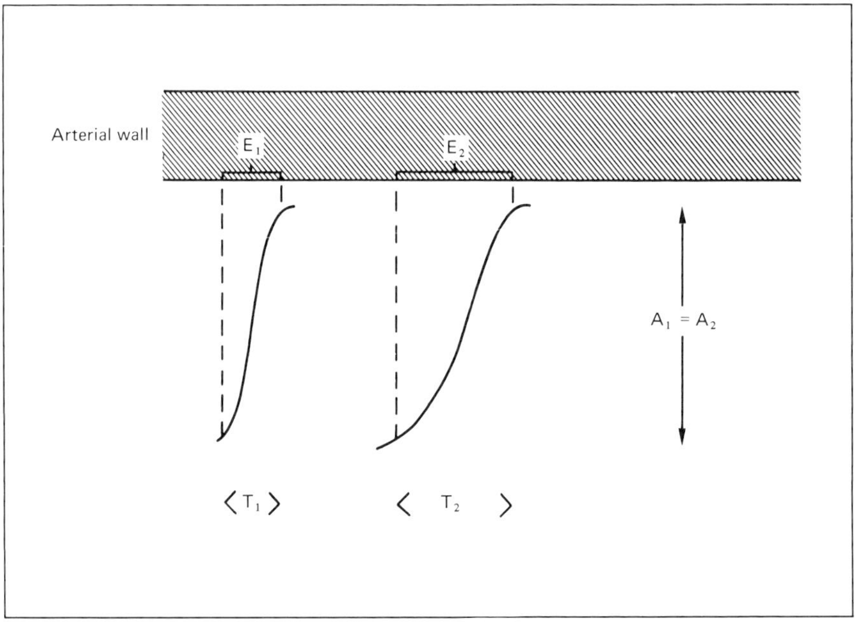

Fig. 1. Relationship between physical energy (E) imparted per area of the arterial wall and the period of the pulse wave (T) at constant pulse pressure [from ref. 72].

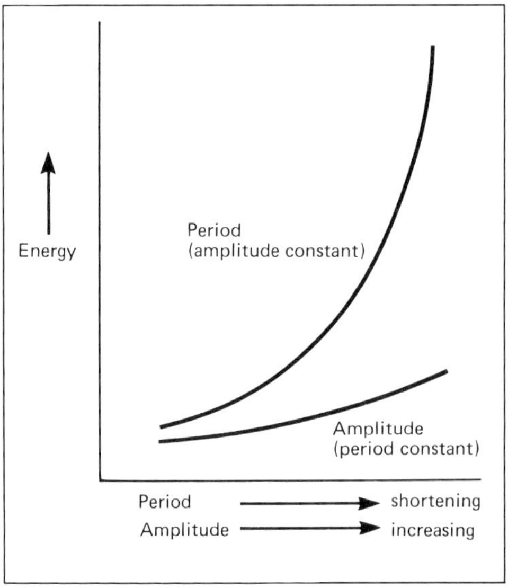

Fig. 2. Idealized relationship between potential energy, period, and amplitude of a pressure wave in a pulsatile system.

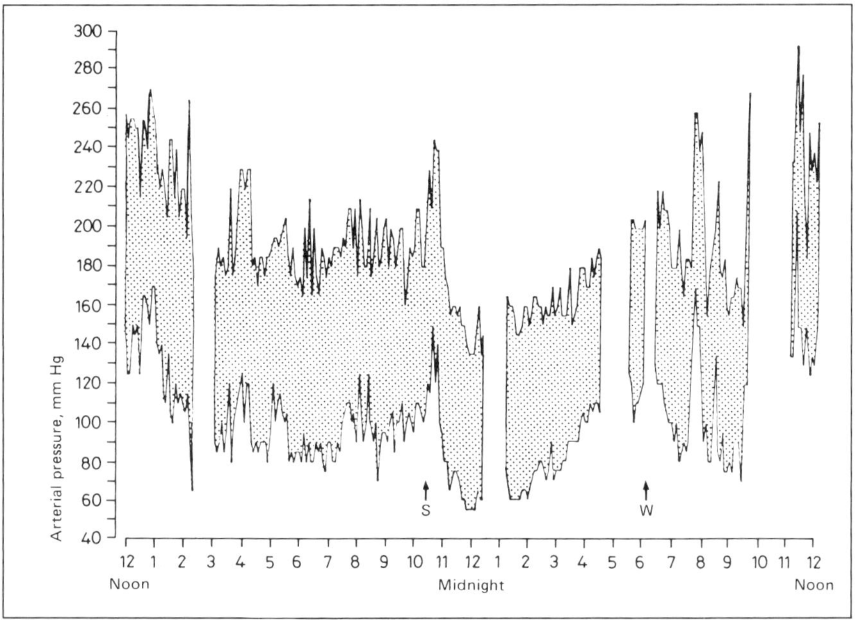

Fig. 3. 24-hour continuous record of arterial blood pressure during normal daily activity in a hypertensive patient. Pressures plotted at 5-min intervals. S = Standing; W = walking [from ref. 52].

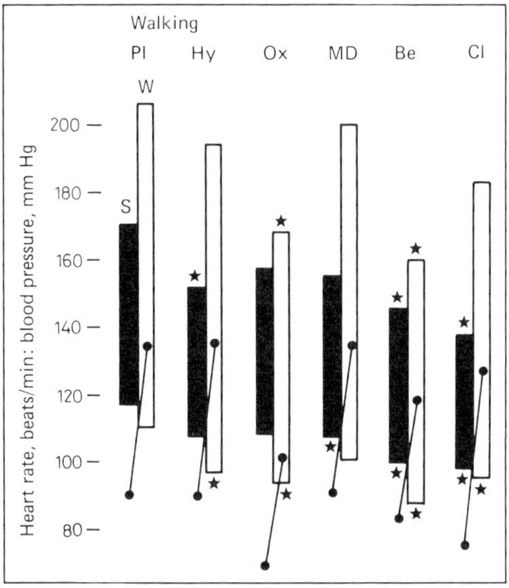

Fig. 4. Crossover comparison of different antihypertensive drugs in suppressing tachycardia and systolic pressor response to dynamic exercise during chronic treatment in 12 hypertensive patients. S = Standing; W = walking; Pl = placebo; Hy = hydrochlorothiazide; Ox = oxprenolol; MD = methyldopa; Be = bethanidine; Cl = clonidine. * $p < 0.05$ compared with placebo response [from ref. 75].

figure 9 of previous chapter). Although beta-blocking drugs have no influence on the hypertensive reaction to cold or isometric exercise – which are alpha-1-adrenoceptor mediated – they do possess two of the three prerequisites for the sensible prevention of precocious coronary artery disease in the hypertensive patient. Furthermore, they are unique among currently available antihypertensive drugs in that they attenuate the oxygen demands on the left ventricle due to increases in heart rate and myocardial contractility. This is important, when it is considered that 1 in 3 patients presenting with high blood pressure already exhibit evidence of ischemic heart disease [11]. The long-term preventive use of beta-blockers in patients with high blood pressure also entails other considerations. Beta-blocking drugs without intrinsic sympathomimetic activity (ISA) result in potentially atherogenic changes in the lipoprotein cholesterol fractions during their long-term administration to hypertensive patients [15, 26, 39, 65, 69]. Beta-blocking drugs with ISA also appear to result in a lesser incidence of side effects, e.g., cold extremities [57, 63, 77] and reduced exercise capacity [16], which may influence patient compliance and nullify the preventive effectiveness of these drugs during long-term treatment. For these reasons, a potent beta-blocking drug with ISA, such as oxprenolol, holds considerable preventive promise in the treatment of hypertension.

Primary Prevention Studies

There is considerable circumstantial evidence in the literature indicating that the cerebrovascular and renal hazards of high blood pressure, but not of coronary heart disease, are reduced by antihypertensive treatment [10, 22, 78, 79]. None of these early, small-scale studies specifically involved beta-blocking drugs. Later, others that did suggested that beta-blocking drugs may prove beneficial in reducing the risk of coronary heart disease in hypertensive patients [8, 38, 64]. The unique and potentially arterioprotective pharmacodynamic activity of beta-blocking drugs taken in conjunction with their secondary preventive potential in nonhypertensive patients stimulated a number of large-scale, long-term primary preventive studies with these drugs. The major studies underway at present are designed to test the influence on morbidity and mortality of oxprenolol, propranolol, or metoprolol, when these drugs are incorporated into conventional antihypertensive regimens in patients with mild or moderate hypertension. For ethical reasons, none involves direct comparison with placebo.

The International Prospective Primary Prevention Study in Hypertension has included 6,700 patients with a diastolic blood pressure of 100–125 mm Hg [30]. In this study patients first receive either oxprenolol, 160–320 mg in a slow-release formulation, or placebo on a randomized double-blind basis. Other conventional antihypertensive drugs are then added, if necessary, to each treatment schedule to lower diastolic blood pressure to less than 95 mm Hg. Entry to the study is now closed, and all patients are being followed for 3–5 years. The results of this study are still awaited, but the excellent overall control of blood pressure in all patients included bodes well for their overall prognosis.

It must be emphasized, however, that it is still unknown whether beta-blocking drugs specifically convey protection against the development of precocious coronary heart disease, compared to other treatments. But the frequency with which coronary heart disease presents in patients with hypertension underlines the potential importance of the results of these primary prevention studies for therapeutic practice.

Prophylactic Modification of Personality Type A Behavior Pattern

The Pavlovian school first alerted medical attention to the potentially untoward cardiovascular consequences of persistent psychic stress in the experimental animal. *Selye* [60, 61] extended these observations into a broad general concept of stress-induced disease. *Friedman and Rosenman* [18] were instrumental in applying such general considerations to the specific coronary hazards of high-arousal states in man. Thus arose the concept that certain psychological and behavioral patterns carried an increased risk of a pathological coronary event [58]. There is now overwhelming evidence that the incidence of coronary events and sudden death is significantly greater in individuals with 'type A' personality/behavior characteristics [59]. This high-arousal state is characterized by an excessive sense of time urgency, punctuality, and impatience; such individuals are also ambitious, competitive, and aggressive. In contrast, the coronary risk is much less in their more easygoing peers (type B). This thesis has received ample, independent confirmation from numerous epidemiologic studies [25, 27, 33, 36, 82]. Individuals with a type A behavior pattern have a twofold excess of coronary heart disease [36]. In men this predilection tends to be concentrated in the more sedentary, but in women there is no such distinction [25]. In both sexes it is independent of other risk factors and other psychosocial markers. The risk attached to a type A behavior pattern is also substantially increased in the presence of the other 'standard' risk factors such as high blood pressure, hyperlipidemia, and so on. Moreover, both folklore and clinical observation have long related sudden death to immediately preceding psychological trauma. Doubts continue to be expressed regarding the causal relationship between personality behavior type and the risk of coronary death [14, 54], but these ignore an impressive array of evidence. Controversy regarding the precise 'diagnostic' definition of the individual at risk has now been largely resolved [34, 55]. Debate has also surrounded the psychosomatic mechanisms involved. The psychological pathways are clearly defined. Psychic stress, whether of endogenous or exogenous origin, results in sympathetic stimulation of the cardiovascular system over well-defined autonomic pathways [43, 71]. Likewise, there is little doubt of the electromechanical mechanisms by which a fatal arrhythmia may arise [71]. Psychological stress greatly reduces the threshold for ventricular fibrillation, even in the normal heart of the experimental animal [44]. In man the frequency of ventricular ectopic beats is clearly related to catecholamine surges and other evidence of increased sympathetic drive [41, 49]. Type A individuals have the same resting blood pressure and catecholamine levels as type B individuals, but they react to psychic stress with exaggerated responses of both [12, 19, 49, 51]. It is thus easy to see the chain of events which may result in electrical death of the heart. The therapeutic implications are also clear. The final terminals through which such stimuli may induce electrical death are the beta-adrenoceptors in the heart, and beta-blocking drugs afford the only pharmacologic remedy protecting the heart from the surges in blood pressure and catecholamine stimulation [71].

Debate has also recently arisen regarding the extent of coronary disease in type A individuals. Many patients who die suddenly have advanced coronary artery disease [42], while many others do not. Unfortunately, information with regard to the relative prevalence of severe coronary artery disease in relation to behavior patterns is relatively scarce. *Heller* [27] found that men who had sustained a myocardial infarction had significantly higher type A scores than did age-matched controls. Some studies of patients with chest pain have described more angiographically demonstrable coronary atheroma in those with type A than in those with type B behavior patterns [9, 17, 81, 83]. Others have been unable to confirm this [3, 13]. The discrepancy results from small, often retrospective analyses that have only clouded the issue. Moreover, these disclaimers of an association between the behavior pattern and extent of coronary atheroma in an individual do not really question the undoubted relationship between the specific behavior pattern of the type A individual and his proneness to myocardial electrical death.

What is the possible explanation of the proneness of the type A individual to coronary death? Epidemiologic studies with ambulatory ECG monitoring have clearly shown that a high frequency of ectopic beats increases the risk of sudden coronary death [28, 40, 41]. This is due to the precipitation of ventricular fibrillation in almost all instances [53]. These latter authors, in a large number of patients resuscitated from a lethal arrhythmia, were also able to demonstrate the neural trigger of the arrhythmia in the myocardium in 50% of patients without evidence of organic heart disease, compared to a similar trigger in only 25% of patients with clinical evidence of coronary disease. This may afford an explanation of the discrepancies in some of the published studies between the incidence of coronary atheroma in type A individuals.

These arguments strongly implicate the role of sympathetic stimulation of the fibrillatory-prone heart as the potential psychophysiologic mechanism relating the risk of coronary death to the behavior pattern of the individual. It is equally rational to suggest that attenuation of the repetitive and exaggerated peaks of hazardous sympathetic influences in the type A individual may best be achieved by blockade of beta-adrenoceptors in the heart. No large-scale studies have as yet been reported to confirm or deny such a suggestion. But such a preventive method would be far less cumbersome in the majority of communities than by trying to modify behavior patterns by other therapeutic techniques [20, 50].

In the absence of such definitive studies can the possible effects of beta-blocking drugs on the coronary risk of type A individuals be predicted from current knowledge of their effects in other closely related clinical situations? Regardless of the psychic origins of stimulation of the midbrain vasomotor center, whether they are caused by excessive alertness and mental drive (type A), endogenous anxiety or excessive exogenous psychic stress, the final common autonomic pathway is over the sympathetic outflow. The final effector terminals in the heart are the beta-adrenoceptors controlling heart rate and myocardial contractility. The myocardial oxygen-wasting results of sympathoadrenal stimulation carry a significant hazard of ischemia and electrical instability in the coronary-prone heart [43, 49, 68, 71]. Beta-blocking drugs effectively attenuate such potentially hazardous stimuli, even in small doses. Oxprenolol has been clearly shown, in many studies, to be preeminent in this respect [66, 67, 70, 73]. The drug has been shown to suppress the unwanted sympathetic stimulation of the heart in many situations associated with excessive mental stress [31, 32, 37, 62, 67, 70, 73]. It has also been shown to be particularly efficacious in suppressing the somatic symptoms associated with emotion and anxiety [21, 24, 46]. Will oxprenolol similarly attenuate the risk beneficially in the coronary-prone individual? Probably yes. Although up to the present time no beta-blocking drug has been tested in this important field of primary prevention, the theoretical and pragmatic considerations outlined above suggest that of the drugs likely to protect the heart effectively in the coronary-prone type A individual, the beta-blockers, including oxprenolol, head the list of contenders.

Secondary Prevention following Myocardial Infarction

In view of the efficacy of beta-adrenoceptor antagonists in reducing the oxygen demands of the ischemic heart, their possible value in preventing the further development of coronary heart disease after myocardial infarction has long attracted clinical interest. Fortunately, the influence of treatment on the prognosis of myocardial infarction lends itself to practical clinical evaluation. The disease syndrome has a definable onset, and its presence is confirmable by objective means. Many myocardial infarction patients are referred to special units, so that standardized methods of diagnosis and care may be practised. Finally, most patients eventually succumb to the further consequences of the disease, thereby facilitating the interpretation of morbidity and mortality data.

Many of the early studies appeared to yield a negative answer in terms of benefit conveyed by these drugs in this condition [5]. Many, however, did not fulfil adequate clinical trial standards (e.g., randomized allocation to double-blind treatment), and most did not fulfil the statistical criteria necessary to substantiate the negative claims made. The majority suffered from a type 2 error, i.e., due to inadequate sample size no benefit was demonstrated when benefit may have been present.

More recently a number of well-executed secondary prevention trials involving many thousands of patients confirmed the potential clinical value of beta-blocking drugs in preventing the subsequent consequences of myocardial infarction [45, 76]. One study with metoprolol [29] demonstrated the benefit of intervention within the first few hours of the onset of symptoms, but in most studies beta-blocking drugs were started between 1 and 8 weeks after infarction was confirmed. Eight late-intervention studies have now been reported, and in all but one there was a trend to benefit which was absolute in two, i.e., the 95% confidence limit of the results did not overlap the zero line of no effect [5]. Three of four [1, 2, 56, 80] studies with alprenolol in relatively small numbers of patients demonstrated a reduction in mortality rate. Two studies have been reported with practolol. The smaller one was inconclusive [7], and, although there was a trend to benefit in the larger study [47], this did not achieve the conventional level of statistical significance in terms of mortality. One study with timolol [48] demonstrated a statistically significant reduced risk of reinfarction and sudden death over 2½ years of treatment. One large-scale trial with propranolol [4] also demonstrated similar benefits, although two smaller studies [6, 23] failed to confirm this finding.

Oxprenolol in Secondary Prevention

In view of the potential of beta-blockade to reduce sympathetic stimulation of the ischemic heart and the high tolerability of drugs with ISA, a long-term secondary prevention study with oxprenolol [74] was initiated in 1973. Since the drug is able to prevent surges in sympathetic stimulation of the heart due to psychic stimuli without significant impairment of exercise tolerance, even in relatively small doses [70–73], a dose of 40 mg twice daily was chosen. When the study was designed, it was also unknown at what time following acute myocardial infarction these drugs would be best commenced. Therefore, patients were included between 1 and 90 months after the original coronary event. The results are intriguing. Inclusion of all patients into the analysis on an 'intention-to-treat' basis, irrespective of the time treatment with the drug was started after their infarction, showed no overall benefit for the group as a whole. However, when the results were analyzed according to the time at which the drug was started after infarction, distinctly dissimilar patterns of response became apparent. In patients who started oxprenolol between 1 and 4 months after infarction, there was a progressive benefit compared to placebo-treated patients which extended for up to 6 years, even when analyzed on a pragmatic intention-to-treat basis (fig. 5). In a similar number of patients included between 5 and 12 months after their infarct, there was no appreciable benefit of active treatment (fig. 6). In neither of these groups did withdrawal from oxprenolol constitute a hazard. In the third group of patients included between 1 and 7

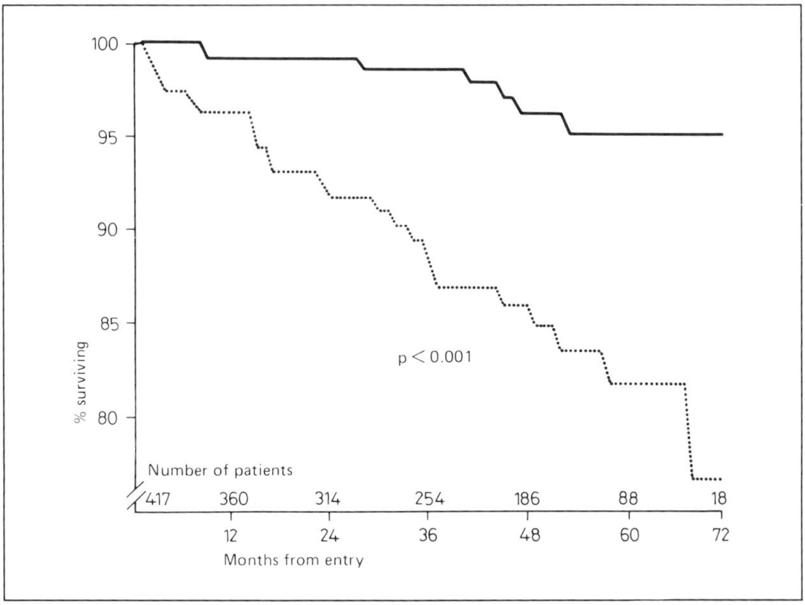

Fig. 5. Life table cumulative survival curves for patients entered within 4 months of infarction. Values are expressed as mean ± SE (bars). —— = Oxprenolol; ··· = placebo [from ref. 74].

years after infarction, oxprenolol appeared detrimental to survival (fig. 7). Closer examination of this latter group, however, reveals that there was an increase in mortality risk only in patients who stopped active treatment; those who continued treatment had a similar benefit to those who started the drug earlier (fig. 8). It is also intriguing that the average time at which most of the deaths occurred in patients withdrawn from active treatment after late (1–7 years) entry was concentrated to more than 2 years after they stopped treatment. Was this a catching-up phase after the earlier mortality risk was delayed? Until randomized stopping procedures at the end of such studies are accepted as ethical tools, this question cannot be answered.

The study with oxprenolol was unique in a number of respects: (1) not only was a similar benefit apparent when the drug was started at a similar time to beta-blockers in other secondary prevention trials, but the benefits persisted for more than 6 years, far longer than has been demonstrated in

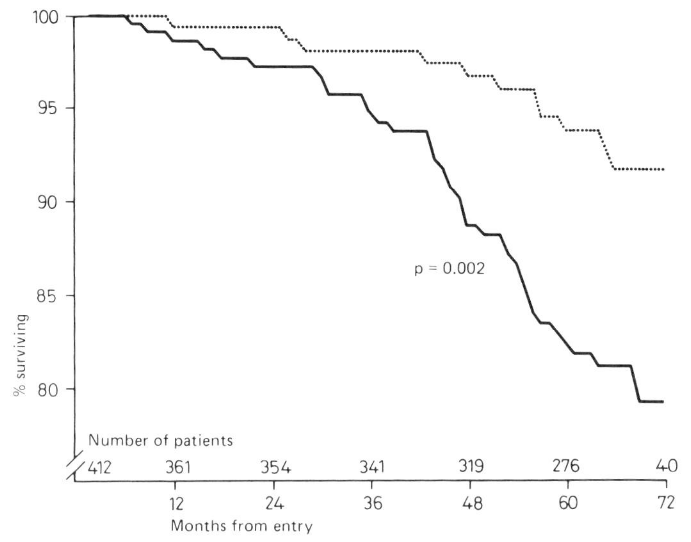

Fig. 6. Life table cumulative survival curves for patients entered more than 12 months after infarction. Values are expressed as mean ± SE (bars). —— = Oxprenolol; ··· = placebo [from ref. 74].

previous studies; (2) the preventive value of the drug was apparent in all patients who continued to take it; (3) stopping the drug in patients in whom it was started *late* after infarction (a group not previously studied) demonstrated a delayed mortality risk, and (4) there was a lower yearly side-effect rate in this study than was reported in other secondary prevention studies with beta-blocking drugs, despite the fact that patients were followed for more than twice as long as those in other studies.

What conclusions may be drawn regarding the value of beta-blocking drugs, and oxprenolol in particular, in the secondary prevention of the further consequences of acute myocardial infarction? Despite the many thousands of patients studied in many clinical trials, overall results of the secondary prevention studies are difficult to apply directly to most survivors of myocardial infarction met under routine circumstances. The survivors met in open clinical practice include an infinite number of subgroups with an immensely wide band of cardiovascular risk factors. It is unreasonable to

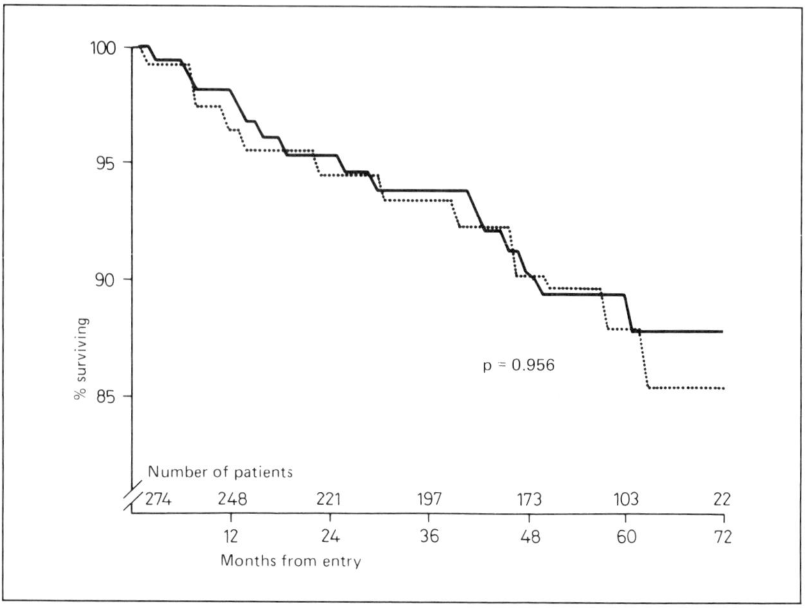

Fig. 7. Life table cumulative survival curves for patients entered between 5 and 12 months after infarction. Values are expressed as mean ± SE (bars). —— = Oxprenolol; ··· = placebo [from ref. 74].

expect that beta-blocking drugs will be efficacious in every subgroup of survivors; in fact, they may even be harmful in some.

Which patient, then, should the physician treat? On the evidence available, it would be reasonable to prescribe these drugs to both male and female patients under 70 years of age in whom their previous infarct has given rise to no serious cardiac complication, e.g., heart failure, heart block, and so forth. Treatment should be started during the convalescent phase and continued for a period of years. Cardioprotection appears to be a general property of beta-blocking drugs, but the withdrawal of these drugs in postinfarction patients may carry both early and long-term hazards. Patient compliance with treatment, therefore, appears to be a vital factor in the benefits offered by these drugs. As this depends on the frequency of adverse reactions, whether of physiologic or other origin, both the dose of drug used and its clinical tolerability are of prime importance in ensuring the continuation of sustained treatment. In these respects oxprenolol is of value.

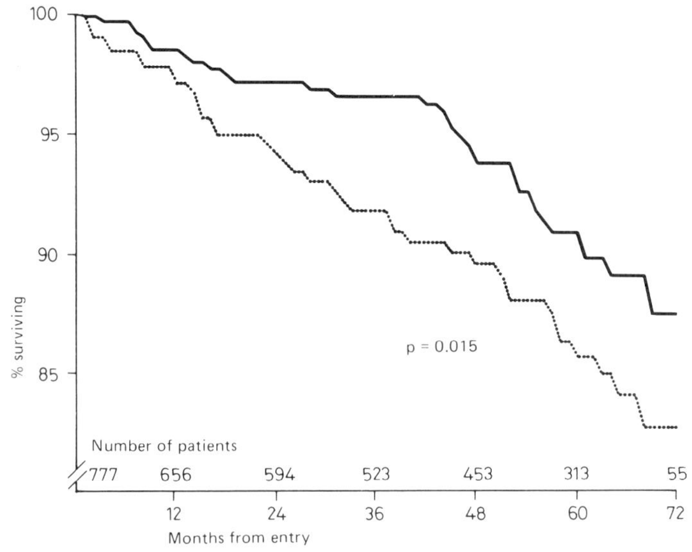

Fig. 8. Life table cumulative survival curves for all patients continuing on allocated trial medicine. Values are expressed as mean ± SE (bars). —— = Oxprenolol; ··· = placebo.

Summary

High blood pressure remains the most important risk factor for coronary heart disease susceptible to therapeutic intervention. The major mechanical factors predisposing to arterial trauma in hypertensive patients are related to the hemodynamic results of sympathetic stimulation of the heart. In theory, oxprenolol possesses a particularly suitable pharmacological means of attenuating such potentially hazardous stimuli. At present, no other form of antihypertensive treatment has been shown to reduce the risk of coronary heart disease. Primary prevention studies with oxprenolol have been initiated, and the results are awaited.

There is now overwhelming evidence that the incidence of coronary events and sudden death is significantly greater in individuals exhibiting type A behavior pattern. Whilst type As experience a greater rise in potentially harmful biochemical parameters on the heart in competitive situations, it is easy to understand the role beta-blockers can play in this state of sympathetic overstimulation. Oxprenolol has been shown to be particularly suited to counter the effects of catecholamines on the heart.

Oxprenolol, as with other beta-blockers, possesses the potential qualities necessary to attenuate the further consequences of myocardial ischemia following infarction. Secondary prevention studies have demonstrated a significant reduction in mortality, when oxprenolol is started within the first few weeks after infarction. The studies were unique in demonstrating that benefit in these patients continues for at least 6 years, but that the preventative potential of the drug was lost when started in patients some years after the acute event. Oxprenolol plays potentially an important role both in the primary and secondary prevention of coronary heart disease.

References

1 Ahlmark, G.; Saetre, H.; Korsgren, M.: Long-term treatment with beta-blockers after myocardial infarction. Eur. J. clin. Pharmacol. *10:* 77–83 (1976).

2 Andersen, M.P.; Bechsgaard, P.; Frederiksen, J.; Hansen, D.A.; Jurgensen, H.J.; Nielsen, B.; Pedersen, F.; Pedersen-Bjergaard, O.; Rasmussen, S.L.: Effect of alprenolol on mortality among patients with definite or suspected acute myocardial infarction. Lancet *ii:* 865–868 (1979).

3 Bass, C.; Wade, C.: Type A behaviour: not specifically pathogenic? Lancet *ii:* 1147–1149 (1982).

4 Beta-Blocker Heart Attack Research Group Trial: A randomized trial of propranolol in patients with acute myocardial infarction. I. Mortality results. J. Am. med. Ass. *247:* 1707–1714 (1982).

5 Baber, N.S.; Lewis, J.A.: Confidence in results of beta-blocker postinfarction trials. Br. med. J. *284:* 1749–1750 (1982).

6 Baber, N.S.; Wainwright-Evans, D.; Howitt, G.; Thomas, W.; Wilson, C.; Lewis, J.A.; Dawes, P.M.; Handler, K.; Tuson, R.: Multicentre post-infarction trial of propranolol in 49 hospitals in the United Kingdom, Italy and Yugoslavia. Br. Heart J. *44:* 96–100 (1980).

7 Barber, J.M.; Boyle, McC.; Chatuverdi, N.C.; Singh, N.; Walsh, M.J.: Practolol in acute myocardial infarction. Acta med. scand., suppl. 587, pp. 213–219 (1975).

8 Berglund, G.; Wilhelmsen, L.; Sannerstedt, R.; Hansson, L.; Anderssen, O.; Sivertsson, R.; Wedel, H.; Wikstradn, J.: Coronary heart disease after treatment of hypertension. Lancet *i:* 1–4 (1978).

9 Blumenthal, J.A.; Williams, R.B.; Long, Y.; Schanberg, S.M.; Thompson, L.W.: Type A behaviour pattern and coronary atherosclerosis. Circulation *58:* 634–639 (1978).

10 Breckenridge, A.; Dollery, C.T.; Parry, E.H.O.: Prognosis of treated hypertension. Changes in life expectancy and causes of death between 1952 and 1967. Q. Jl Med. *39:* 411 (1970).

11 Dawson, J.R.; Sutton, G.C.: Detection of clinically significant coronary artery disease in hypertensive patients. Echocardiographical study. Br. Heart J. *46:* 595 (1981).

12 Dembroski, T.M.; MacDougall, J.M.; Herd, J.A.; Shields, J.L.: Effects of level of challenge on pressor and heart rate responses in type A and B subjects. J. appl. soc. Psychol. *9:* 209–228 (1979).

13 Dimsdale, J.E.; Hackett, T.P.; Hutter, A.M.; Block, P.C.; Catanzano, D.M.; White, P.J.: Type A behaviour and coronary angiographic findings. J. psychosom. Res. *23:* 273–276 (1979).

14 Editorial: Are we killing ourselves or not? Lancet *ii:* 669–670 (1981).

15 England, J.D.F.; Simons, L.A.; Gibson, J.C.; Carlton, M.: The effects of metoprolol and atenolol on plasma high-density lipoprotein levels in man. Clin. exp. Pharmacol. Physiol. *7:* 329–333 (1980).
16 Franciosa, J.A.; Johnson, S.M.; Tobian, L.J.: Exercise performance in mildly hypertensive patients. Impairment by propranolol but not oxprenolol. Chest *78:* 291–299 (1980).
17 Frank, K.A.; Heller, S.S.; Kornfield, D.S.; Sporn, A.A.; Weiss, M.B.: Type A behaviour pattern and coronary angiographic findings. J. Am. med. Ass. *240:* 761–763 (1978).
18 Friedman, M.; Rosenman, R.H.: Association of specific overt behaviour pattern with blood and cardiovascular findings; blood cholesterol level, blood clotting time, incidence of arcus senilis and clinical coronary artery disease. J. Am. med. Ass. *169:* 1286–1296 (1959).
19 Friedman, M.; Byers, S.O.; Diamant, J.; Rosenman, R.H.: The plasma norepinephrine response of coronary-prone subjects (type A) to a specific challenge. Metabolism *24:* 205–210 (1975).
20 Friedman, A.: The modification of type A behaviour in post-infarction patients. Am. Heart J. *97:* 551–560 (1979).
21 Gosling, R.H.: Clinical experience with oxprenolol in the treatment of anxiety in the United Kingdom; in Kielholz, Beta-blockers and the central nervous system, pp. 125–130 (Huber, Bern 1977).
22 Hamilton, M.; Thompson, E.N.; Wisniewski, T.K.M.: The role of blood pressure control in preventing complications of hypertension. Lancet *i:* 235–238 (1964).
23 Hansteen, V.; Moinichen, E.; Lorentsen, E.; Andersen, A.; Strom, O.; Soiland, K.; Dyrbekk, D.; Refsum, A.-M.; Tromsdal, A.; Knudsen, K.; Eika, C.; Bakken, J., Jr.; Smith, P.; Hoff, P.I.: One year's treatment with propranolol after myocardial infarction: preliminary report of Norwegian multicentre trial. Br. med. J. *284:* 155–160 (1982).
24 Hawkins, J.R.: Clinical experience with beta-blockers in consultant psychiatric practice. Scott. med. J. *20:* 294–298 (1975).
25 Haynes, S.G.; Feinleib, M.; Kannel, W.B.: The relationship of psychosocial factors to coronary heart disease in the Framingham Study. III. 8 year incidence of coronary heart disease. Am. J. Epidem. *3:* 37–48 (1980).
26 Helgeland, A.; Hjerman, I.; Leren, P.; Enger, S.; Holme, I.: High-density lipoprotein cholesterol and anti-hypertensive drugs: the Oslo Study. Br. med. J. *ii:* 403–404 (1978).
27 Heller, R.F.: Type A behaviour and coronary heart disease. Br. med. J. *ii:* 368 (1979).
28 Hinkle, L.E.; Argyros, D.C.; Hayes, J.C.; Robinson, T.; Alonso, D.R.; Shipman, S.C.; Edwards, M.E.: Pathogenesis of unexpected sudden death. Role of early cycle ventricular premature contractions. Am. J. Cardiol. *39:* 873–879 (1977).
29 Hjalmarson, A.; Elmfeldt, D.; Herlitz, A.; Holmberg, S.; Malex, I.; Nyberg, G.; Ryden, L.; Svedberg, K.; Vedin, A.; Waagstein, F.; Waldenstrom, A.; Waldenstrom, J.; Wedel, H.; Wilhelmsen, L.; Wilhelmsson, C.: Effect on mortality of metoprolol in acute myocardial infarction. Lancet *ii:* 823–827 (1981).
30 IPPPSH Collaborative Group: The International Prospective Primary Prevention Study in Hypertension – objectives, design and preliminary data review; in Burley,

Birdwood, The clinical impact of beta-adrenoceptor blockade, pp. 193–203 (Ciba, Horsham 1980).

31 James, I.M.; Pearson, R.M.; Griffith, D.N.W.; Newbury, P.: Effect of oxprenolol on stage-fright in musicians. Lancet *ii:* 952–954 (1977).

32 James, I.M.; Pearson, R.M.; Griffith, D.N.W.; Newbury, P.; Taylor, S.H.: The effect of oxprenolol on stress-induced disturbances of performance. Proc. R. Soc. Med. *70:* suppl. 11, p. 34 (1977).

33 Jenkins, C.D.: Recent evidence supporting psychological and social risk factors for coronary disease. New Engl. J. Med. *294:* 987, 1033 (1976).

34 Jenkins, C.D.: Estimation of the coronary-prone behavior pattern by use of the structured interview and the activity survey; in Rosenman, Psychosomatic risk factors and coronary heart disease: indications for specific preventative therapy, pp. 22–28 (Huber, Bern 1982).

35 Kannel, W.B.; Dawber, T.R.: Hypertension: a cardiovascular risk profile. Br. J. Hosp. Med. *2:* 904–911 (1974).

36 Kannel, W.B.: Established cardiovascular risk factors – Framingham today; in Kielholz, Siegenthaler, Taggart, Zanchetti, Psychosomatic cardiovascular disorders – when and how to treat?, pp. 69–96 (Huber, Bern 1981).

37 Krishnan, G.: Oxprenolol in the treatment of examination nerves. Scott. med. J. *20:* 288 (1975).

38 Lambert, D.M.D.: Long-term survival on beta-receptor blocking drugs in general practice; in Burley, Birdwood, Fryer, Taylor, Hypertension – its nature and treatment, pp. 283–289 (Ciba, Horsham 1975).

39 Lehtonen, A.; Viikari, J.: Long-term effect of sotalol on plasma lipids. Clin. Sci. *57:* 405S–407S (1979).

40 Lown, B.; Calvert, A.F.; Armington, R.; Ryan, M.: Monitoring for serious arrhythmias and high risk of sudden death. Circulation *52:* suppl. 3, pp. 189–198 (1975).

41 Lown, B.; Tempt, J.V.; Reich, P.; Caughan, C.; Regestein, O.; Hai, H.: Basis for recurring ventricular fibrillation in the absence of coronary heart disease and its management. New Engl. J. Med. *294:* 623–629 (1976).

42 MacKinnon, A.; Taylor, S.H.: Relationship between 'sudden' coronary deaths and drinking water hardness in 5 Yorkshire cities and towns. Int. J. Epidemiol. *9:* 247–251 (1980).

43 Malliani, A.: Central and reflex regulation of the sympathetic nervous system and psychosomatic cardiovascular disorders; in Kielholz, Siegenthaler, Taggart, Zanchetti, Psychosomatic cardiovascular disorders – when and how to treat?, pp. 59–63 (Huber, Bern 1981).

44 Matta, R.J.; Verrier, R.L.; Lown, B.: The repetitive extrasystole as an index of vulnerability to ventricular fibrillation in the dog. Am. J. Physiol. *230:* 1469–1473 (1976).

45 May, G.S.; Eberlein, K.A.; Furberg, C.D.; Passamani, E.R.; DeMets, D.L.: Secondary prevention after myocardial infarction: a review of long-term trials. Prog. cardiovasc. Dis. *24:* 331–352 (1982).

46 Michael, J.: A placebo-controlled double-blind trial of oxprenolol versus diazepam in the treatment of anxiety and stress; in Kielholz, Siegenthaler, Taggart, Zanchetti, Psychosomatic cardiovascular disorders – when and how to treat?, pp. 191–196 (Huber, Bern 1981).

47 Multicentre International Study: Improvement in prognosis of myocardial infarction by long-term beta-adrenoceptor blockade using practolol. Br. med. J. *iii:* 735–741 (1975).
48 Norwegian Multicentre Study Group: Timolol-induced reduction in mortality and reinfarction in patients surviving acute myocardial infarction. New Engl. J. Med. *304:* 801–807 (1981).
49 Orth-Gomer, K.: Evidence of psychological influence on the formation of ventricular arrhythmias: implications for preventive therapy; in Rosenman, Psychosomatic risk factors and coronary heart disease: indications for specific preventive therapy, pp. 42–48 (Huber, Bern 1983).
50 Patel, C.: Yoga and biofeedback in the management of 'stress' in hypertensive patients. Clin. Sci. mol. Med. *48:* 171S–174S (1975).
51 Perini, C.; Muller, F.; Buhler, F.R.: Personality; coronary prone behaviour and adrenergic factors in hypertension; in Rosenman, Psychosomatic risk factors and coronary heart disease: indications for specific preventive therapy, pp. 37–41 (Huber, Bern 1983).
52 Pickering, G.: High blood pressure (Churchill, London 1981).
53 Reich, P.; DeSilva, R.; Lown, B.; Murawski, B.: Acute psychological disturbances preceding life-threatening ventricular arrhythmias. J. Am. med. Ass. *246:* 233–235 (1981).
54 Joint Working Party of the Royal College of Physicians of London and the British Cardiac Society: Prevention of coronary heart disease. J. R. Coll. Physns *10:* 213–275 (1976).
55 Review Panel on Coronary-Prone Behaviour and Coronary Heart Disease: Coronary-prone behaviour and coronary heart disease, a critical review. Circulation *63:* 1199–1215 (1981).
56 Reynolds, J.L.; Whitlock, R.M.I.: Effects of a beta-adrenergic receptor blocker in myocardial infarction treated for one year from onset. Br. Heart J. *34:* 252–259 (1972).
57 Roberts, C.J.C.; Marshall, A.J.; Barritt, D.W.: A study of cold extremities in patients taking beta-blocking drugs; in Judd, Topics in cardiovascular disease, pp. 168–179 (Ciba, Horsham 1976).
58 Rosenman, R.H.; Brand, R.J.; Jenkins, C.D.; Friedman, M.; Strauss, R.; Wurm, M.: Coronary heart disease in the Western Collaborative Group Study. Final follow-up experience of 8½ years. J. Am. med. Ass. *233:* 872–877 (1975).
59 Rosenman, R.: Coronary-prone behaviour pattern and coronary heart disease: implications for the use of beta-blockers in primary prevention; in Rosenman, Psychosomatic risk factors and coronary heart disease: indications for specific preventive therapy, pp. 9–14 (Huber, Bern 1983).
60 Selye, H.: A syndrome produced by diverse noxious agents. Nature, Lond. *139:* 32–33 (1963).
61 Selye, H.: Stress and cardiovascular disease. Cardiovasc. Med. *4:* 183–191 (1979).
62 Siitonen, L.; Janne, J.: Effect of beta-blockade during bowling competitions. Ann. clin. Res. *8:* 393–398 (1976).
63 Smith, R.S.; Warren, D.J.: Effect of acute oral beta-adrenergic blockade on muscle blood flow in man. Cardiovasc. Res. *16:* 205–208 (1982).
64 Stewart, I.Mc.D.G.: Compared incidence of first myocardial infarction in hyperten-

sive patients under treatment containing propranolol or excluding beta-receptor blockade. Clin. Sci. mol. Med. *51:* suppl. 3, pp. 509–512 (1976).
65 Streja, D.; Mymin, D.: Effect of propranolol on HDL cholesterol concentrations. Br. med. J. *ii:* 1495 (1978).
66 Taggart, P.; Carruthers, M.: Suppression by oxprenolol of adrenergic response to stress. Lancet *ii:* 256–258 (1972).
67 Taggart, P.; Carruthers, M.; Sommerville, W.: Electrocardiogram, plasma catecholamines and lipids and their modification by oxprenolol when speaking before an audience. Lancet *ii:* 341–346 (1973).
68 Taggart, P.; Carruthers, M.: Emotional stress-induced arrhythmias. Proc. R. Soc. Med. *70:* suppl. 11, pp. 41–43 (1977).
69 Tanaka, N.; Sakaguchi, S.; Oshige, K.; Niimura, T.; Kanehisa, T.: Effect of chronic administration of propranolol on lipoprotein composition. Metabolism *25:* 1071–1075 (1976).
70 Taylor, S.H.; Meeran, M.K.: The cardiovascular response to some environmental stresses and their modification by oxprenolol; in Burley, Fryer, Rondel, Taylor, New perspectives in beta-blockade, pp. 293–306 (Ciba, Horsham 1973).
71 Taylor, S.H.: Stress, cardiovascular disease and beta-adrenoceptor antagonists; in Kielholz, Beta-blockers and the central nervous system, pp. 90–108 (Huber, Bern 1977).
72 Taylor, S.H.: Stress, hypertension and ischaemic heart disease; in Kielholz, Siegenthaler, Taggart, Zanchetti, Psychosomatic cardiovascular disorders – when and how to treat?, pp. 120–137 (Huber, Bern 1981).
73 Taylor, S.H.; Meeran, M.K.: Different effects of adrenergic beta-receptor blockade on the heart rate response to mental stress, catecholamines and exercise. Br. med. J. *ii:* 257–259 (1973).
74 Taylor, S.H.; Silke, B.; Ebbutt, A.; Sutton, G.C.; Prout, B.J.; Burley, D.M.: A long-term prevention study with oxprenolol in coronary heart disease. New Engl. J. Med. *307:* 1293–1301 (1982).
75 Taylor, S.H.; Taylor, J.A.; Watt, S.J.; Swaby, M.J.: Drug prevention of pressor responses in hypertensive patients; in Yamori, Lovenberg, Freis, Perspectives in cardiovascular research, pp. 409–414 (Raven Press, New York 1979).
76 Turi, Z.G.; Braunwald, E.: The use of beta-blockers after myocardial infarction. J. Am. med. Ass. *249:* 2512–2516 (1983).
77 Vandenburg, M.J.; Conlon, C.; Ledingham, J.M.: A comparison of the effects of propranolol and oxprenolol on forearm blood flow and skin temperature. Br. J. clin. Pharmacol. *11:* 485–490 (1981).
78 Veterans Administration Cooperative Study Group on Antihypertensive Agents: Effects of treatment on morbidity in hypertension. I. Results in patients with diastolic blood pressure averaging 115–129 mm Hg. J. Am. med. Ass. *202:* 1028 (1967).
79 Veterans Administration Cooperative Study Group on Antihypertensive Agents: Effects of treatment on morbidity in hypertension. II. Results in patients with diastolic blood pressure averaging 90–114 mm Hg. J. Am. med. Ass. *213:* 1143 (1970).
80 Wilhelmsson, C.; Vedin, A.; Wilhelmsen, L.; Tibblin, G.; Werko, L.: Reduction of sudden deaths after myocardial infarction by treatment with alprenolol. Lancet *ii:* 1157–1161 (1974).

81 Williams, R.B.; Harey, T.; Gentry, W.D.; Kong, Y.: Relation between hostility and arteriographically documented coronary atherosclerosis in type A and non-type A patients. Psychosom. Med. *40:* 88–96 (1978).
82 Zyzanski, S.J.: Coronary-prone behaviour pattern and coronary heart disease: epidemiological evidence; in Dembroski, Weiss, Shields, Haynes, Feinleib, Coronary-prone behavior (Springer, New York 1978).
83 Zyzanski, S.J.; Jenkins, C.D.; Ryan, T.J.; Flessas, A.; Everist, M.: Psychological correlation of coronary angiographic findings. Archs intern. Med. *136:* 1234–1237 (1976).

S.H. Taylor, University Department of Cardiovascular Studies and Department of Medical Cardiology, The General Infirmary, Leeds (England)